The Writing Diet

By Julia Cameron

BOOKS IN THE ARTIST'S WAY SERIES

The Artist's Way

Walking in This World

Finding Water

The Complete Artist's Way

The Artist's Way Workbook

OTHER BOOKS ON CREATIVITY

The Writing Diet

The Right to Write

The Sound of Paper

The Vein of Gold

The Artist's Way Morning Pages Journal

The Artist's Date Book, *illustrated by Elizabeth Cameron*

How to Avoid Making Art (or Anything Else You Enjoy)
    illustrated by Elizabeth Cameron

Supplies: A Troubleshooting Guide for Creative Difficulties

Inspirations: Meditations from *The Artist's Way*

The Writer's Life: Insights from *The Right to Write*

The Artist's Way at Work *(with Mark Bryan and Catherine Allen)*

Money Drunk, Money Sober *(with Mark Bryan)*

The Writing Diet

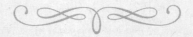

WRITE YOURSELF
RIGHT-SIZE

Julia Cameron

JEREMY P. TARCHER/PENGUIN

a member of Penguin Group (USA) Inc.

New York

JEREMY P. TARCHER/PENGUIN
Published by the Penguin Group
Penguin Group (USA) Inc., 375 Hudson Street, New York, New York 10014, USA ·
Penguin Group (Canada), 90 Eglinton Avenue East, Suite 700, Toronto, Ontario
M4P 2Y3, Canada (a division of Pearson Canada Inc.) · Penguin Books Ltd,
80 Strand, London WC2R 0RL, England · Penguin Ireland, 25 St Stephen's Green,
Dublin 2, Ireland (a division of Penguin Books Ltd) · Penguin Group (Australia),
250 Camberwell Road, Camberwell, Victoria 3124, Australia (a division of Pearson Australia
Group Pty Ltd) · Penguin Books India Pvt Ltd, 11 Community Centre, Panchsheel Park,
New Delhi–110 017, India · Penguin Group (NZ), 67 Apollo Drive, Rosedale,
North Shore 0632, New Zealand (a division of Pearson New Zealand Ltd) ·
Penguin Books (South Africa) (Pty) Ltd, 24 Sturdee Avenue,
Rosebank, Johannesburg 2196, South Africa

Penguin Books Ltd, Registered Offices: 80 Strand, London WC2R 0RL, England

First trade paperback edition 2008
Copyright © 2007 by Julia Cameron

Most Tarcher/Penguin books are available at special quantity discounts for bulk purchase for sales
promotions, premiums, fund-raising, and educational needs. Special books or book excerpts also can
be created to fit specific needs. For details, write Penguin Group (USA) Inc. Special Markets, 375
Hudson Street, New York, NY 10014.

The Library of Congress catalogued the hardcover edition as follows:

Cameron, Julia.
The writing diet : write yourself right-size / Julia Cameron.
p.   cm.
ISBN 978-1-58542-571-6
1. Weight-loss—Psychological aspects.   2. Creative writing.   I. Title.
RM222.2.C257   2007   2007022970
613.2'5—dc22

ISBN 978-1-58542-698-0 (paperback edition)

Printed in the United States of America
1   3   5   7   9   10   8   6   4   2

Book design by Meighan Cavanaugh

Neither the publisher nor the author is engaged in rendering professional advice or services to the
individual reader. The ideas, procedures, and suggestions contained in this book are not intended as
a substitute for consulting with your physician. All matters regarding your health require medical
supervision. Neither the author nor the publisher shall be liable or responsible for any loss or damage allegedly arising from any information or suggestion in this book.

While the author has made every effort to provide accurate telephone numbers and Internet ad-
dresses at the time of publication, neither the publisher nor the author assumes any responsibility
for errors, or for changes that occur after publication. Further, the publisher does not have any control over and does not assume any responsibility for author or third-party websites or their content.

This book is dedicated to my beloved mother,

who suffered both from being overweight and from many

dark depressions about it. These struggles impaired

her ability to lead a creatively fulfilling life.

I loved her dearly and miss her deeply.

Author's Note

Please note: The names of people discussed and quoted in *The Writing Diet* have been changed to protect their privacy. In some cases composite characters have been used. All such alterations have been made for the purpose of simply condensing concepts I have often observed. It is my hope that this book will help you lead a healthier and more creative life.

Contents

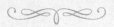

Part Two

SITUATIONS AND SOLUTIONS

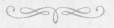

Prologue

THE WRITING DIET

I'm a creativity expert, not a diet expert. So why am I writing a book about weight loss? Because I have accidentally stumbled upon a weight-loss secret that works. For twenty-five years I've taught creative unblocking, a twelve-week process based on my book *The Artist's Way.* From the front of the classroom I've seen lives transformed—and, to my astonishment, bodies transformed as well. It took me a while to recognize what was going on, but sure enough, students who began the course on the plump side ended up visibly leaner and more fit. What's going on here? I asked myself. Was it my imagination, or was there truly a "before" and an "after"? There was!

To my seasoned eye, weight loss is a frequent by-product of creative recovery. Overeating blocks our creativity. The flip side is also true: we can use creativity to block our overeating. That is what we will be doing with this book, using creativity tools to attack our overweight, altering our weight through altering our consciousness. Believe it or not, writing is a weight-loss tool—overlooked, underused, and extremely powerful.

It's not as if I've never tried traditional dieting. On the contrary—I'm an amateur expert. Over the years I've tried Atkins, but my cholesterol zooms; South Beach, but I gain back everything the minute I veer away from phase one; the Gray Sheet from Overeaters Anonymous, but deprivation makes me crazy and crazy is what I am trying to avoid as well as fat. I've turned myself in to Weight Watchers, but counting points seems to be its own form of craziness. What I know how to count is words. In building twenty-plus books, I have learned that each word counts, just like each calorie. Suddenly—literally—I have food for thought. What if words can be consumed instead of calories? What if I can write my way right-size? As soon as the idea hits me, I know in my marrow that it is true.

Everyone knows that we overeat because something is eating us. What if that question got asked directly, routinely, every time we ate? What if, struck by a Snack Attack, I said to myself, "What's eating me that I have a sudden craving to eat?" What if I took a moment and jotted down my feelings? What if I gave myself food for thought instead of food itself? Since we can use food to block feelings, why can't we use words to block food? Calories, after all, are units of energy, and so are words.

This idea excites me. Long experience as a writer has taught me that writing is a way to metabolize life. If I can write about something, I can handle it—and often with grace. Might writing be a way to metabolize the ebb and flow of my very metabolism? I think it might. I was never thin, nor was I ever fat—not until I had to take a medication that lists weight gain as a possible side effect. The medication is a necessity. The weight gain is, to my doctor's eye, a small price to pay for mental stability. Surely, I think, there must be some way out. Could it be writing?

In the twenty-five years I have taught creative unblocking, one of the tools I routinely teach is daily morning writing. How often have I seen my students use their Morning Pages to shed pounds as well as creative inhibitions? Although in an Artist's Way class what we are after is a creative renaissance, a physical renaissance often goes with it, hand in glove. Students often come to me pudgy and depressed. I tell them to write. A steady diet of self-reflection soon regulates their overeating. Pounds begin to drop away. As their Morning Pages work to metabolize their lives, they no longer overeat to block their difficult feelings. Their creativity soars while their weight drops. From the front of the classroom, the transformation is often startling.

Laura, a kindergarten teacher, began her creative unblocking, frankly, overweight.

A tall, still-beautiful blonde, she carried an extra forty pounds on her frame. She dressed in slimming black, but the illusion that she was thin was unconvincing. Laura was the kind of woman of whom it was routinely said, "It's a shame she's so heavy. She has such a pretty face."

The survivor of a violent childhood home, Laura had learned early to block her feelings with food. Writing her daily Morning Pages, she began to face her turbulent feelings. As she did, the urge to block her emotions with food began to melt away. The pounds melted away too, and Laura emerged from a twelve-week course a far slimmer swan of a woman. She attributes her weight loss to her writing. "There were so many little things bugging me," she recalls. "My Morning Pages were gripe sessions where I saw and worked out my grudges." Once she found out what was eating her, she no longer needed to overeat.

Writing makes us conscious. Once we are conscious, it is difficult to act out in unconscious ways. Once we catch on that we are overeating as a blocking device, it becomes harder to reach for food and easier to reach for words. That is what this book teaches you to do. When a Snack Attack hits, you can take yourself to the page instead of to the refrigerator. When you do, your creativity will respond with an increased flow of insights and ideas.

"It was right on the tip of my tongue," we often say when an idea eludes us. What we don't realize is that ideas often do live right on the tip of our tongue—and that we drown those ideas when we overeat. Michael, a writer, reports that when he snacks on sweets and starches, his writing dries up, but when he eats a healthful snack like a piece of fruit, the flow of his writing surges forward. Mary Alice, another writer, reports that when she writes down her feelings, she is rewarded by an increased flow of creative power. "It is as though when I name one thing I am given the names for many other things," she says.

Our emotions become known to us. Known, they are no longer the saboteurs causing us to overeat. All of us are creative and all of us can be more creative than we are. As we relinquish our blocking devices, we come into our power. In this book we are specifically focusing on food as a blocking device—and on writing as a means to weight control.

WHAT TO EXPECT

Although many of my students report that they have found new and exciting lives after following my creativity work, I cannot promise you a new career if you undertake the Writing Diet. What I can promise you is increased clarity, increased energy, increased productivity. As you write, you will lose weight and gain creativity. As you unblock your feelings, you will gain access to the energy that they hold. As you become more familiar with yourself, the origin of your creative work, you will become, quite literally, more original. As you become more lean, your thinking will grow more clear. As you lose weight, you will stop waiting for the magic wand that will transform your life. Instead, you will realize that the magic wand is actually a pen and that, pen in hand, you can transform your own life.

Unlike most diet books that proclaim that they alone have the answer, the Writing Diet works successfully with any sensible eating plan. Writing is the key. You can write on Atkins. You can write on South Beach. You can write on Weight Watchers and Overeaters Anonymous. In fact, using the tools of the Writing Diet will greatly increase your chances of success with whatever diet you choose.

If you are drawn to this book, odds are good that you feel you are both creative and creatively stifled. You literally hunger for a more satisfying life. Working with the tools of the Writing Diet can give you that life. Your sweet tooth will be satisfied by the sweet satisfaction of a richer and more fulfilling life.

For simplicity's sake, this book is divided into two parts. Part

One introduces you to seven simple tools. They are the bedrock of your recovery from overeating. Part Two features essays on the many situations and circumstances you may find yourself facing. Each of these essays is paired with a further tool that will deepen your consciousness and creativity.

Part One

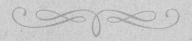

THE TOOLS

The First Tool:
Morning Pages

*T*he first tool of the Writing Diet is a tool I have taught many times before. It is the basic tool of creative unblocking and the basic tool of successful long-term weight loss as well. You will write three pages every morning, a practice that I call Morning Pages. They are to be strictly stream of consciousness, no "high art" here. You simply move your hand across the page and write whatever thought comes into your head. Even "non-thoughts" are fine. Don't expect or demand that you have a writing style. Any style at all will do. So fret, gripe, worry, scold—or celebrate. There is no wrong way to do Morning Pages.

Your pages may sound grumpy and whiny—"I'm awake and I want to sleep two more hours. I hate my job. I hate my boss. I hate the life I have invented for myself these days." Your pages might sound anxious and scattered. You might find yourself angry or sad. It's all right. It's all all right. Your job is simply to get down on the page whatever it is you are.

What you are doing with your pages is something that in 12-step parlance is called "getting current." You are out to catch up on yourself, to pinpoint precisely what you are feeling and thinking. It's an interesting phrase, "getting current." Because that is exactly what we are doing. We are tapping into the energy flow in our lives, the current of who and what we are. When I get current, I feel more alive. I know who I am and what I want more of and what I want less of. Writing Morning Pages, I tap into a creative energy that flows like a subterranean river through my life.

One of the first fruits of Morning Pages is an upsurge of creativity in many forms. Apartments get painted. Curtains get hung. Long-overdue letters get written. Art forms that we have lost or forgotten come wafting back to us with increased urgency. "Don't put me off any longer," these zephyrs beg. When we listen to them, we start to flourish.

Morning Pages galvanize our days. They prioritize them as well. Writing Morning Pages, we begin to see that each day is made up of myriad "choice points" and that we have a great deal of freedom to choose exactly how we will live. Morning Pages make us aware of which activities are dead ends for us and which activities give us a sense of health and well-being. Like a tough-love friend, Morning Pages nudge us in the direction of needed change.

"I really need more exercise," we write one day. And a second day. And a third. On the fourth day we abruptly realize that we can take a twenty-minute walk on our lunch hour. We take that walk and the next day's pages record this small triumph.

Morning Pages put us in touch with our emotions. Often those emotions have been clogged, stuffed down beneath the weight of our busy days, days filled with work, relationships and, yes, food. Too often we have touched our feelings and recoiled as from a hot stove. We have been angry and felt our anger was taboo. We have been sad and turned to some mindless television to ignore it. We have even turned to food when we felt joy. Any intense emotion can trigger a Snack Attack.

Writing Morning Pages, our mindless lives are behind us. A day at a time, a page at a time, we become mindful, acutely attuned to our personal feelings. We might write ".I am angry at my sister. Talking with her bores me silly. She just gets me on the phone and does a monologue. We haven't had a real conversation in years!" Realizing how we feel, we often make spontaneous changes. To our needy sister we say, "Wait a minute—there's something I want to tell you"—and then we tell her that we are not a wailing wall and that she, too, needs to learn to listen. To our surprise, she hears us. For the first time in years, conversation is a two-way street.

The pages examine all of our relationships, not the least of which is our relationship to food. "The junk food I am eating leaves me hungover," we might write. The very next day, faced with an opportunity to binge, we decline. "What's come over you?" our friends ask as we order a salad Niçoise instead of our usual chicken potpie.

"My tastes have changed," we might joke, but more than just our tastes are changing. Jeannie began her day on Coca-Cola and moved on from there to Cheerios. "It was like a five-year-old was feeding me," she laughs. Her Morning Pages pointed out to her that she was living on sugar and starch and that a few fruits and vegetables might be in order. One day she found herself buying a container of fresh strawberries. "I've always loved fresh strawberries, but I never let myself have them. I just didn't feel deserving. A month of pages changed the habits of years. I simply couldn't bear to see how I was treating myself. Once I did see it, I knew it had to stop—and it did."

The last time I heard from Jeannie, strawberries were a staple in her diet. She had exchanged her morning Coca-Colas for tea and had even started making herself salads for lunch. She had dropped three dress sizes and lost the telltale bloat on her fine-featured face. In the photo that she sent of herself and her new boyfriend, she looked fifteen years younger than her pre-pages self.

Morning Pages sweep the house of our consciousness. They poke into every odd corner of our thoughts. They are a catcher's mitt for many small ideas that lead to larger breakthroughs. "I'd like this room better red," we think one day of the foyer to our apartment. A week later the room is red and we do, in fact, like it better. But now we think our living room could use some sprucing up. It looks so dull by comparison. . . .

A day at a time, a room at a time, we remake our environment. Now our apartment looks like someone with self-worth lives there. And someone with self-worth is struggling to be born.

"This relationship is suffocating me," we might write. Cornered by our pages, we face the difficult fact that our marriage is arid and that we feel parched and exhausted from trying single-handedly to make it work. "I deserve reciprocity," we scrawl early one morning. Later in the day we tell the same thing to our spouse. Standing up for ourselves, we begin to walk taller. We feel the self in self-worth.

It takes courage to undertake Morning Pages, but pages themselves give us courage. In the privacy of our journal, we admit the secrets we have been harboring. Once aired, those secrets lose their power to tyrannize us. Our pen is the scalpel with which we lance the psychic infections we have been carrying. "I hate this job," we write. "It's prestigious, but there's too much stress for too little reward."

Once we target a problem area, the pages are quick to suggest solutions. We are not trapped, pages remind us. We always have choices. Sometimes those choices are difficult. We may hate our job but love our salary. Pages encourage us to take accurate stock of our situation. Perhaps, for right now, the job is worth all its aggravation. We can choose to leave or we can choose to stay. Pages help us to sort our options.

Many of us find, writing pages, that we seem to be put into contact with a source of wisdom greater than ourselves. Answers swim into consciousness that seem far wiser than our personal thinking. It is for this reason that I have come to think of Morning Pages as an effective form of meditation—especially for hyperactive Westerners. Most of us have a hard time with conventional meditation. It is very difficult for us to sit calmly and do nothing for twenty minutes. With pages, you sit calmly and do something. That something, the motion of the hand across the page, is actually a way of tracking what meditators speak of as "cloud thoughts." As our thoughts cross our consciousness, we record them on the page. Oddly, the very act of writing down our concerns helps us to put those concerns in their proper perspective. We miniaturize our irrational worries. We underscore our legitimate concerns. Morning Pages are a sorting process. At first on the page and then in our lives, we begin to get things straight.

With our pages as our ally, we begin to face down difficult issues. Some of us face squarely a long-suspected drinking problem. Others admit to using television as a potent narcotic. Many of us find that food is our favored blocking device.

"I was a late-night eater," says Anthony. "I didn't realize this until I began to record in my Morning Pages what felt like hang-overs. I wasn't drinking. In fact, I prided myself on several years of sobriety, but there was no question that my mornings were hungover and that food was the substance I was abusing."

Self-knowledge is often the first step toward change, and when Anthony admitted his abusive eating, he took a step toward discontinuing it. "It didn't happen overnight," he says. "But I began to record, 'hungover again,' and then, one night, I aborted a late-night snack halfway through, saying to myself, 'You don't want to be hungover in the morning, do you?' "

When Anthony abandoned his late-night binges, he found that he had immediate access to greater creative energy. "I found I was full of late-night ideas and that a fear of this energy had been at the root of my overeating." No longer overeating to thwart his creativity, Anthony saw that he had many healthy choices in front of him. For one thing, he had the time and energy to write his long-delayed memoirs.

"My extra pounds were a barricade I placed between me and my freedom," he realized. "When I gave up late-night grazing, the pounds slowly began to slip away and I found myself making many healthy changes."

Believing himself trapped in a dead-end job, Marcus saw that he was in fact unwilling to do the footwork to find new employment. He was in jail, all right, but he held the key—he just needed the will to use it.

"One morning, I wrote 'I hate my job' for the last time," he recalls. "That day I picked up the phone and called a head hunter. I soon learned that I was eminently employable."

Morning Pages point us in the direction of our growth. They make us intimate with ourselves and that, in turn, allows us to be more authentically intimate with others. Leslie found herself writing that she was unhappy in her relationship. As she explored this in subsequent pages, she learned that she was hungry for deeper communication than what she enjoyed with her lover. "Try telling him that," her pages suggested one morning. The advice brought Leslie face-to-face with the fact that she had almost sabotaged her relationship rather than risk honesty within it.

As we risk honesty in our pages, it becomes easier to be honest elsewhere. Leslie admitted in her Morning Pages that she was feeling stifled by her lover's codependency. "I resented his possessiveness, but I also went along with it because I was, frankly, a little flattered by it," she says. In her pages she rehearsed what she wanted to say: "I just need a little more breathing room," she told him. "I don't want to do everything together." When she risked more disclosure, he risked more disclosure in turn. To her surprise, he admitted to similar feelings. They were actually both feeling smothered. This conversation gave them the courage to open the cage door. They soon found that their increased independence gave their time together greater intensity and meaning.

Greater intensity and meaning are common experiences for those who choose to work with Morning Pages. The experience is not unlike falling in love—but the object of our affections is now the Self. We become interesting to ourselves. Our thoughts, feelings, and perceptions count for something. A page at a time, a day at a time, we are becoming intimate with ourselves, and that intimacy is often both threatening and thrilling.

Janice undertook Morning Pages because of a mysterious

malaise that she did not understand. She was happily married to Bill, a charismatic, high-powered salesman. He spoiled her with material blessings. Her every wish was his command. Every year Bill's earning power seemed to increase. They traded in home after home, always moving to bigger and better abodes. Pampered and pudgy, Janice dutifully decorated each new nest—but she resented it.

Janice's pages suggested to her that their pursuit of the great American Dream was actually a frenzied and empty pursuit. "I didn't need more. I actually needed less. I needed to be able to cherish what I had, not constantly trade it in for something else." With the help of pages, Janice saw that her own dreams had become submerged beneath the dreams and goals of her husband. She wanted to write—and more than the steady stream of bread-and-butter notes that their lifestyle demanded. Bill traveled in his work. Janice was often lonely, but she decided to use her empty time to take a writing course. Her creativity took off like a rocket. Soon she was asked to script a radio show—then to host it.

"I became a writing fiend," Janice laughs. "They were paying me to write, but I would have paid them!" She also became thinner, no longer an overstuffed hen sitting on her nest egg.

Morning Pages teach us what we like—and what we don't like. A line at a time, they move us closer to our authentic selves. In Morning Pages we stop hiding. We come out into the open—at least on the page. "I'd really like to try . . ." we write—and then we try it. Dreams long deferred move, step by step, into reality. We discover that as we move our hand across the page, a Higher Hand moves across the surface of our lives. For many of us, pages are a spiritual experience as we make contact with a Power Greater Than Ourselves.

Alice lost both of her parents to early deaths. An adult, she often still felt like an orphaned child. She was surprised to find comfort in writing Morning Pages. Time and again she would write out guidance that seemed to her far wiser than any of her own devising. "At first it was as if I became my own wise parent. Then I began to wonder if perhaps my own parents weren't speaking to me through the pages. They began to feel much closer to me and I began to feel far less alone. The pages became for me a source of companionship and strength. I began to think of them as my personal spiritual practice. They kept me on track and gave me an even keel."

For many of us, an even keel is elusive. We long for stability but we do not know how to find it. Pages may be the first effective form of mentoring that we encounter. We make contact with what might be called an Inner Mentor. Under its tutelage, we are able both to remain stable and to take risks.

Alan began doing Morning Pages when he took an Artist's Way class. For twelve weeks he wrote every morning, watching with some awe as his ordinary life became transformed. For many years he had dreamed of being a playwright. At the urging of pages he now tried a few short monologues—and read them aloud to great success at an open mic. With such encouragement, you might think he would be firm in keeping to his new regimen— instead, when his class ended, Alan abandoned it.

As Alan abandoned his pages, he abandoned himself. No longer listening for guidance, he accepted a new, high-powered job in a field that he didn't really like. In fact, the only thing to like about his new job was the salary. Frustrated and a little ashamed of himself, Alan began to overeat. He kept a steady supply of snack foods in his desk drawer at the office, and whenever his conscience bothered him, he reached for a treat. Before he realized what had happened, Alan had packed on twenty-five pounds. Always a big man, he was now too big. When Alan and I crossed paths, I suggested he go back to his Morning Pages to see if he could determine what was eating him and why he found it necessary to overeat.

"I don't know why I ever quit," Alan quickly reported. Within three weeks of being back on the page his eating patterns began to come under control. He no longer treated his desk like an extension of his refrigerator. "I really hate this job," he admitted. "I think I sold myself out to take it."

At the urging of his pages, Alan turned in his resignation, determined to find new work that was more in accord with his value system. He also began writing again, and one more time his monologues met with public success.

"I think I have a knack for this," Alan told me modestly. I suggested he find a day job that left him with enough energy to pursue his writing in the evenings. Before long Alan was offered a job that seemed perfect to him. He believed in the company and its goals and he found that working along the lines of his true values didn't stress or tire him the way his old, toxic job had. No longer conflicted, Alan found that he could both work his day job and write in the evenings. Before long he found the courage to tackle a full-length play—a dream that had for years eluded him.

"I think I learned my lesson," Alan now says. "I need the honesty and self-reflection that Morning Pages afford me. I am not a spiritual man, but I seem to be living now along more spiritual lines. I find I like it."

"I find I like it" may be for most people the bottom line in working with Morning Pages. As we vent our anxieties, our stresses, and our frustrations, a new equanimity begins to take hold. We feel different and we begin to look different.

"What did you have," the joke runs, "a face-lift or a surrender?"

I began working with Richard during the worst months of a long, cold New York winter. A blocked Broadway actor, he carried an extra thirty pounds. It was his "insulation," he joked, but to me the weight wasn't a laughing matter. It was creative suicide. When I looked at Richard, I saw the handsome leading man struggling to emerge. His diet of pizza and cheeseburgers and Entenmann's chocolate chip cookies was pure sabotage. I put him on a regimen of morning writing and fairy tales. (Yes, fairy tales.)

Against his better judgment, Richard began Morning Pages. He quickly saw his own negative patterns. He overworked. He overate. Fatigued and frustrated, he undernurtured himself. Pizza became the panacea for his misery. He had big dreams and a bigger waistline, but the closest he got to Broadway was his favorite pizza stand. He was afraid to take a genuine risk. I suggested he take one on the page. Why not use a fairy tale to bump off a creative monster, someone who had been damaging to his creative self-esteem? Could he think of anyone? He could.

"Fine," I said. "Now write a tale in which you do him in."

"This is really, really stupid," Richard told me, but he went home and wrote a fairy tale about a former music teacher. In the fairy tale the teacher suffered a fate worse than death—he always sang off-key. Richard was jubilant that his abusive former teacher had finally gotten his comeuppance. Sharing the fairy tale with the class, his glee was contagious.

"Good for you," I told Richard. "Now what?"

Richard flushed. "Actually, there is a now-what," he admitted. "I've signed up for voice lessons and I've given up cookies, pizza, and cheeseburgers with everything."

The last I heard of Richard, he had dropped twenty of his unwanted pounds, gotten new head shots taken, and was auditioning again.

From the front of the classroom, the transformation that Morning Pages causes is almost startling. Even after two and a half decades as a teacher, I am still struck with wonder as people seem to change right before my eyes. I call the process "spiritual chiropractic" as changes are made in exactly the direction that they are needed. Overeaters curb their binges. Undereaters begin to eat more regularly. From the front of the room, the increased health is readily evident. And "all" they are doing is writing.

Writing "rights" things. Dead-end jobs are abandoned. Ditto for dead-end relationships. Energy is spent along new and more productive lines. Dreams that were elusive begin to seem possible. As we become increasingly unblocked, our lives flourish. As we become more fit, our lives become more fitting. At age forty-five Deanna embarked on law school. At age fifty James went back for a master's in poetry. Georgianna did the same thing at seventy-five. In each case, their morning writing led them into more adventurous and expanded lives.

Much to their surprise, people get happy when they write. Once we get used to it, writing is as natural as breathing—and almost as necessary. Moving our pen across the page, we come into focus to ourselves. Emotions long avoided become familiar. Perceptions become clearer. Boundaries begin to fall in place. Guided by our own hand, without years of costly therapy, we begin to break our unhealthy patterns and dependencies. We become true to ourselves—and more true to others.

"Thank you for Morning Pages. My husband is a far happier man," a woman told me. I have heard this sentiment many times over the years.

"I thought I needed a divorce," admits Kevin. "What I really needed was a way for me to take responsibility for my own happiness."

Morning Pages are a route to happiness. For many people that happiness is expressed as weight loss.

TASK

Write Your Morning Pages

This tool is the bedrock of creative recovery. It will challenge you, enrich you, and enliven you. Set your clock an hour early, although you may not need that much time. Take yourself to the page and report precisely how you are feeling. Nothing is too petty or too large to be included. Keep your hand moving and follow your thoughts. They may be quite fragmented and scattered. That's all right. Do not expect "real" writing. Just let yourself write. There is no wrong way to do Morning Pages. They are for your eyes only. Let yourself write. Remember—and trust—that you will be able to write yourself right-size.

The Second Tool:
The Journal

You will write your Morning Pages daily, but you will write far more often than in the mornings. Throughout your day, you will write every single time you eat—and every single time you feel like eating. This tool is not about judgment. It is about accuracy. Many of us do not know exactly what we eat on a given day. We become discouraged because we gain weight despite our best efforts to the contrary. Keeping a food journal takes the guesswork and wishful thinking out of our lives. Instead, we have facts. We know what we ate, and as we become more skilled at using our journal, we know why we ate it. It is simple and straightforward. You will write down every morsel you eat. You will write down what you are feeling when you are tempted to eat. Very often you will find that you are eating instead of taking a creative action. The creative action does not have to be big. It may be something simple like cleaning up your room. It may be something harder like making a difficult phone call. Whatever the action is, you will often find that you eat to blur your clarity and avoid action. Stunned by a sugar high, who can say precisely what needs to be done next? How many times has a pint of Ben and Jerry's replaced an action in your life?

Weight loss is a process. At its best, it is gradual and gentle—so gentle, it is almost imperceptible. One day, "suddenly," we are thinner. Our clothes fit more loosely. We have more energy. We feel more ourselves. We have lost weight and we have often done it after repeated, unsuccessful attempts to do it. We have finally found the right something or somethings that help us to chisel off the pounds.

The something that works for me and my students is words. We put language between us and a binge. We put language on our turbulent emotions. We name our inner landscape, and that process of accurate self-definition is exciting. To do this, we keep a journal, although it records far more than our eating—or our battle not to eat. At the first whisper of a Snack Attack, we take to the page. Pen in hand, we explore our troubling cravings. "I want to eat something," we write. And then we keep on writing. Revelations tumble to the page.

Whenever and whatever we are tempted to eat, we record.

"I want to eat something" soon translates into something far more specific. For example, "I just thought of John, and that made me want to stuff my feelings of loss. I still miss John." Or "This new job is exciting but so public that I find it a little threatening."

As we admit the shadows that fall across our inner terrain, those shadows lose their power to scare and to sabotage us. We can live with missing John, we can live with the stress of the new job—and we can do it without a pint of ice cream.

Not all of the feelings that drive us to the cookie cabinet are negative. Sometimes good news sends us spinning. Working with pages and journaling, Andrew lost ten pounds and was so elated by the news from his scale that he went on an eating binge to celebrate—and sabotage—his loss. "I had to laugh," he says, "although it wasn't funny. Using the tools, I managed to nip myself mid-binge. I told myself it was progress, not perfection."

Stress triggers self-defensive eating and stress can come from new positives in our lives as well as from old negatives. We may "still" miss John, but it is equally likely that our new, higher-profile job makes us nervous and that those nerves also give us a Snack Attack.

"I had a best-selling book and suddenly everyone wanted my picture," one author relates ruefully. "I was finally in a position to 'show them' and what I showed them was that I'd packed on fifteen pounds on a book tour. My new designer suits were too tight and my 'cute little face' looked pudgy. I wanted to scream."

Faced with self-sabotage, we all want to scream, but we can do something far more productive. We can write. First thing in the morning, we can do our Morning Pages. At midday, instead of reaching for an oversize lunch, we can reach for our journal and in it we can record the facts and feelings of the day. "I am at the hairdresser's. They are sending out for Chinese. I am tempted, but I think I'll skip it," Marjorie wrote. She asked for—and got—a Starbucks coffee and a salad instead.

Although, at first, journaling may feel foreign and intrusive, it soon becomes a natural and indispensable source of companionship and courage.

Caitlin found she used her journal to say the unsayable. A teacher of gifted students, she frequently found their parents to be obnoxious and spoiled—unlike their offspring, whom she thoroughly enjoyed. And so, faced with a parent-teacher meeting, she scrawled in her journal, "I hate and resent these meetings. These parents treat me like the downstairs maid. I can't stand it!" Venting her pent-up negativity, Caitlin found herself able to skip the high-calorie buffet laid out for the parents' visit. No Brie and crackers for her. No gorgonzola with apple. No chocolate chip cookies. No New York cheesecake. Nothing but clarity.

"I felt so good, facing my true feelings. I also found that venting my feelings gave me room for other feelings, more positive feelings. As I wrote in my journal after the meeting was over, 'That wasn't so bad.' "

Speaking for myself, my journal became a constant companion, a best friend to whom I confided my innermost thoughts—especially when I was on the road working. Reaching for my journal instead of for food, I found that I had a whole range of feelings that I had previously not acknowledged.

I discovered that I overate at lunch on book tours because I was often bored by yet another hotel room, and the day seemed "too long" to me. As I was writing my feelings in my journal, it occurred to me that a really good book might be the antidote to my lunchtime blues. I decided to make my room service lunch secondary to the adventure of what I was reading. I would read something delicious instead of eating. I chose a romantic novel by Tim Farrington, The Monk Downstairs. I couldn't wait to get at it every day. I found I had a larger appetite for Farrington's words than I did for an overinflated lunch. Journaling taught me that I was using food out of boredom and that when I wasn't bored, I wasn't hungry.

Writing in his journal, Ned discovered he was genuinely hungry every afternoon at four. "That's when I would grab a bag of chips or a handful of cookies," he relates. "It occurred to me while writing about it that I could bring fruit with me for a snack. Now

I pack some delicious little plums, and when I get a Snack Attack, I eat them."

For Alec, midnight was truly the witching hour. "Every night I would go on an eleventh-hour run," he remembers. "I would race to a fast food chain that closed at midnight. I'd stuff myself with a fast food burger and fries." Writing in his journal, Alec discovered that he became discouraged late at night. No matter how well he had done during the day, as darkness settled in, it settled into his psyche as well.

"Pray," I suggested to Alec. "Pray on the page. Write a prayer."

Dubious at first, Alec began writing out a late-night prayer instead of going on an eating binge. He discovered a whole range of hidden emotions—it was at night that his dreams would come stalking him, urging him to live differently than he was. A successful therapist, Alec had buried his own dreams beneath the dreams of his clients. Artistic by temperament if not career, he had given up piano playing and he had given up writing. At the urging of his journal, he began to take baby steps in each pursuit. He bought a Casio keyboard with earphones that allowed him to play the piano late at night without disturbing his neighbors. Carrying his journal with him at all times, he began to "get" short poems, the first since his college days. Late-night bingeing became a thing of his past.

"I didn't think I'd have the discipline to keep a journal," Brenda reports. "I tried it with a great deal of resistance. What I found out quickly was that keeping a journal made me feel far less lonely. Suddenly I had a witness to my days. It sounds corny, but the journal became my friend."

 "The first journal I bought had horses on the cover," Karen laughs. "Horses made me think of a younger and happier me, one who had a sense of adventure. I quickly found out that journaling also gave me a sense of adventure. 'Someone'—the journal—wanted to know where I went and what I thought. I found myself writing about much more than food."

For many users the journal is a first step toward adventure. Recording our thoughts and perceptions, we find that we are actually far more interesting than we may have thought. Far from boring, our daily lives are fraught with many small dramas. When we put these on the page, a transformation occurs. "Boring old me" becomes "fascinating me." Our largely uneventful lives may unfold like Jane Austen novels, and we are, after all, the heroines and heroes. What we think and feel does matter. As we see that each day is filled with many tiny choice points where we can act and react differently, we begin to respond to life more as we wish to respond to it and less as hapless victims.

"Journaling made me start to see myself as a character—and a character I liked," reports Gillian. "I began to ask myself, 'Would Gillian do that?' when something came up that felt out of sync. I learned that I had a definite style and that this style was something I could further cultivate. Journaling helped me to do that."

"I don't call it a journal. That's too feminine for me," says Matthew. "I call what I write 'field reports,' and I think of them as letters home from the front line. As you might guess, I think of life as an adversarial situation. Part of that is my job as a salesman, which is dog-eat-dog. I discovered from one field report that I ate to cover my feelings of vulnerability. I wanted to be 'big enough' to handle the competition. No wonder I overate."

To Matthew's surprise, his field reports quickly gave him a feeling of inner security. Secure and well grounded thanks to his writing, he no longer found life quite so adversarial. He no longer needed to overeat just to feel right-size.

Liza, too, found that journaling brought her welcome stability. A manic-depressive in her mid-fifties, she was resigned to ping-ponging moods and weight to match. When she was manic, she was too hyper to eat. When she was depressive, she overate. A look at her scale could often tell her accurately where she was in her cycle. As she wrote out her actions and reactions, Liza found herself feeling compassion for herself. So many ups! So many downs! For the first time, she sought the help of a psychophar-macologist. After several tries, they found a medication that gave her access to her emotions yet tempered her erratic mood swings. Her life stabilized, and with it, her weight.

"Journaling makes me smarter," Bob claims. "At the very least it allows me to capture my good ideas before they fade away." An advertising copywriter, Bob uses his journal to brainstorm. "I started out writing about my weight. I would reach for my jour-nal whenever I had a Snack Attack. What I soon discovered was that snacks had been blocking a lot of ideas. When I gave up my Oreo habit, it felt like my IQ jumped up a few points. Instead of munching a cookie, I'd chew over a new idea. I got some of my best campaigns that way."

If journaling can make us thinner and smarter, why don't more people try it?

"I thought journaling was for writers," Patsy says. "And no way was I a writer."

"It seemed so permanent," jokes Carl. "There on the page in black and white. I think I had a fear of commitment. Make that I *know* I had a fear of commitment."

Journaling is not for writers only. A lawyer recently told me, "Journaling has made me a hell of a lot better in the courtroom." Journaling does not require a major commitment—as Carl feared. The only commitment necessary is the commitment to try it. And then try it again the next day.

TASK

Buy Yourself a Journal and Carry It with You Always

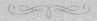

For many of us, this task is an exercise in boosting our self-worth. We are willing to journal, but we go about it in a ragtag fashion, writing on whatever scraps of paper we have at hand. The idea of having a dedicated journal strikes us as spendthrift, too big—and too costly—a commitment. It is not too big a commitment. It is far less costly than the extra pounds you are carrying. Ask yourself, what kind of journal would I like and would I use? Some favor spiral-bound journals that remind them of their schooldays. Others like hardcover journals small enough to fit into their purse. Pick a journal that pleases you and do not be stingy with yourself about the price. Weight loss is worth the cash outlay—and the self-awareness you will gain is beyond price. Carry your journal with you everywhere. Use it whenever you eat—and whenever you want to eat.

The Third Tool:
Walking

Writing brings motion into our lives. A habit of daily Morning Pages brings us into contact with our thoughts and feelings. We learn "what's eating us." From our food journal we learn what we ourselves are eating. This is good as far as it goes, but it doesn't go quite far enough. We need to exercise as well as exorcise our demons. The best way to do so is by walking. I live in Manhattan, a walker's paradise. Stepping out the front door, I can turn right toward a busy street or I can turn left and explore Central Park. I let my feet decide which route to take and then I follow them, curious about where they will lead. They always lead to adventure.

"But, Julia, I don't have time to walk!" you may protest. This is resistance. Resistance tells us we have no time.

None of us has time to walk, not in our hard-driven lives. Walking seems so frivolous. There are the kids, the husband, the career to think about. What's worse, walking seems so time consuming. Where is there time for walking in a life led on the run? Time is what we all need more of—or do we? Twenty minutes a day can be chiseled out of the busiest life simply by replacing our worrying with walking—and walking does help teach us not to worry.

Dorothy, the mother of seven children, felt she had no time to walk. One of her many children always needed her, and when it wasn't her children it was her husband. "I was always 'on call,' " she remembers. "Like a doctor. I couldn't imagine calling a time-out for myself."

"Surely you can manage twenty minutes," I coaxed her.

"No way," Dorothy protested. "If I have a free twenty minutes, I run a load of laundry."

"Five?" I cajoled. "A tiny, miniature, five-minute walkette?"

"Where would I go?" Dorothy demanded to know. "Five minutes isn't long enough to go anywhere!"

"You would go out the front door and then wherever your feet lead you."

"You're trying to trick me, aren't you?" Dorothy protested. "I do that with my kids."

"I am trying to coax you," I responded.

"Oh, all right, but only five minutes, right?"

"Right."

Dorothy remembers, "The hardest part was getting my feet out the door. I had a million excuses to delay myself. And the kids! You would have thought I was going off to India to live in an ashram!" The first time Dorothy made it out the door, we chalked up a V for victory.

"Persistence overcomes resistance," I told her. "Try for five minutes every day."

"We'll see," Dorothy laughed—and we did see.

Before a month had passed, Dorothy's five minutes a day stretched to ten, and before long to a full twenty. She began to cherish her walks and look forward to them. Her weight, stubbornly "stuck," began to slide ever so slightly downward. "I love walking!" she bubbled to me. "I walk out of the house with problems and I walk back in with solutions." She is not alone in this reaction. When I teach creative unblocking, students resist their walks, then fall in love with them. Over the course of a semester, their twenty-minute walks may well stretch toward an hour.

"I learned to enjoy my own company," reports Carole, a recovering bookworm who got her nose out of a book long enough to enjoy the surrounding scenery a step at a time. It was remarkably hard for her to overcome her resistance. Although she wanted to think of herself as an adventurous person, she resisted even the smallest real-life adventure.

"I unkinked my legs and my thoughts," asserts Jay, a graphic designer who finds walks frequently give him creative ideas.

"I de-aged myself," claims Catherine, a sixty-year-old who seems to have shed years as well as pounds.

For many of us, walking brings a sense of heightened vitality and even youth. A step at a time, a calorie at a time, we burn away our lingering malaise and step up our metabolism.

Although we often speak of having a "body of work," we do not often look at the place that "body" occupies relative to our work. We tend to think of creativity as an intellectual construct, something rather disembodied and vaguely "spiritual." This notion is nonsense. Creativity is not something ethereal. It is something very real, an energy that best serves us when it is grounded. And we ground our creativity through our bodies, most easily and most sensibly through walking.

When I lived in Taos, New Mexico, I walked daily amid sagebrush and mountains. Now a Manhattanite, I walk amid the carefully sculpted wildness of Central Park. I enter the park at Eighty-sixth Street, walking down a slight incline toward the glittering reservoir. The trees arch overhead, huge oaks yielding up a bounty of acorns. It is my habit to scoop up pocketfuls of acorns, fingering them like prayer beads as I walk.

I walk daily, stretching my soul as well as my legs. As I walk, I pray for creative guidance. I ask for help on my projects, an intuition as to what direction to move in next. I ask to be made beautiful like the trees are beautiful, each growing according to a unique plan. Lop off a limb and the tree will accommodate its loss, still growing and still beautiful. It is my hope to be able to flourish in similar fashion, taking on the shape and dimension that is intended for me. A creative disappointment may mean a twist in my growth, my life turning in an unexpected direction. As I walk, I pray to grow gracefully, to go along with God's intentions instead of insisting on my own.

When we walk, our problems are drawn to scale. We may set out beleaguered with problems that seem too outsize for us to be able to cope with. A terrible grief may dwarf our steps—but that is only at first. As we walk, our problems fall into a different perspective. As our hearts connect to the Great Creator, our problems seem to diminish. The most terrible losses become bearable. We sense an influx of what might be called grace.

When my father died, I went for long daily walks. My grief

seemed insurmountable, but each day's walk helped to tame it. I would walk a long loop out through the sagebrush, ending at a little creek bed. "I miss my dad," I would sing, a small mourning song, only to suddenly sense that my father was all around me— in the sage, in the red earth, looming above me on the Sacred Mountain. Walking helped my sense of loss give way to a sense of continuity. My sense of dreadful separation gave way to a sense of connection. I would walk out feeling empty, devoid of any creative impulses, and I would walk back home mysteriously replenished, able one more time to sit and to write.

When I teach, I often ask my class how many of them intuitively walk when they are in emotional trouble. More than half the hands shoot up. Walking is a healing tool. We turn to it by instinct. "How many of you know to walk when you are trying to figure something out?" I ask. Again the hands shoot up. "How many of you walk when you are in grief?" More hands. Walking is a self-administered medicine, one that we intuitively know enough to use. What we need to learn is to walk in all times, not merely times of trouble.

Walking can be a conscious tool of inspiration and connection. We do not need to wait for hard times to set out walking. In fact, if we walk often, hard times may become far fewer. Walking miniaturizes our difficulties. Walking, we see things against the scrim of a larger perspective. We sense we are not alone with our problems. There are other, higher forces that guard and guide and comfort us. Walking, we are the recipients of what I call Alpha Ideas, thoughts that seem to come from a higher consciousness than our own, thoughts that are at once simple and bold. I was out walking when it first occurred to me that I could write music—

a seemingly preposterous idea. I was forty-five years old. Surely, if I were musical, I would have known it?

Returning home, I continued to poke at the idea: "Musical? Me?" But the idea, like most Alpha Ideas, was a stubborn one. It did not go away. Instead, it kept returning every time I walked, seeming to garner plausibility with each recurrence. I was out walking in the High Rockies when my first song came to me.

> *My green heart is filled with apples.*
> *Your dark face is filled with stars.*
> *I'm the one that you've forgotten.*
> *You're the one my heart desires.*
> *So dance when you think of me.*
> *Sing to remember me.*
> *Sing till your heart can see*
> *Who we are. . . .*

Hearing this melody and the words, I dashed back up the mountain to my girlfriend's house, where I quickly sang the song into a tape recorder. Next, I sang the song for my girlfriend and her husband. They listened, as enchanted as I was. The melody was beautiful. I had walked into an unexpected talent.

Out walking after that, I began routinely to carry a tape recorder, hoping to be able to "catch" other songs. Sure enough, other songs came to me. They came to me when I was not walking, but they came most often when I was. To me, this seemed nothing short of miraculous. I had grown up as the official non-musical sibling in a highly musical household. Music was something I had always aspired to but not something I thought I could create. Walking taught me otherwise.

"It was while I was out walking that it came to me to go to graduate school," James relates. "At first I thought the idea was crazy. Where would I ever get the money? I walked some more, and as I walked I realized that people take out school loans and I could do the same even though I was a fifty-year-old man. The more I walked, the more plausible the idea seemed to me. What began as an impossible notion gradually began to seem quite doable. Eventually, I thought, 'Of course I should get my master's!' And I did."

The habit of walking tutors us in the art of intuition. It amplifies what mystics call "the still, small voice." "Solvitur ambulando," St. Augustine observed: "It is solved by walking." When we walk, the two halves of our brains converse.

"I walk out with a question," says Danielle, a young writer, "and after I have been walking for a while I will get a hunch or an urge, 'Call Aunt Sue. Ask her what to do.' In other words, the walking may not provide a direct answer, but it will provide the guidance that leads me to an answer. Sometimes it is literally about just taking the next right step. I may feel stymied or stuck, but if I go for a walk, I usually get direction about what my next move should be. 'Call so and so. Turn left here. Make a right at the corner'—something."

"I think of walking as meditation," asserts Chrissy, a fledgling Buddhist. "When I do my Morning Pages, I am 'sending,' but when I am out on a walk, I am able to receive. I have always had a hard time with sitting meditation. I seem to need to be in motion in order to receive." Zen Master Dogen speaks of this process as "the walking of the self."

It is no accident that walking helps us to receive. Walking tutors us in the art of breathing—and regular, repetitive breath is central to successful meditation. As we walk, our breath becomes more rhythmic. As our breathing stabilizes and deepens, we become more centered. The "still, small voice" becomes more audible.

Honored spiritual traditions recognize this fact. The English walked to Canterbury. The Muslims trek to Mecca. Native Americans pursue vision quests by walking out into the wilderness. Druids and Wiccans walk ley lines in pursuit of spiritual knowledge. In Tibet, the very word for "human" translates as "a goer" or "one who goes on migrations." We can take a cue from these ancient traditions. A habit of walking yields spiritual and creative breakthroughs.

Brenda Ueland, the famed writing teacher, recommended a habit of walking for inspiration "alone and every day." She believed that walking revved the engine of inspiration. Novelist John Nichols walks daily. So does writing teacher Natalie Goldberg. The British Lake poets were all great walkers. (Is it an accident that poetry is divided into "feet"?) Their hours on foot were surpassed only by their output on the page. All of us can increase our outflow by walking. Walking is a surefire path to creativity.

When I teach creative writing, I urge my students to walk. "Plot will come to you and so will character," I tell them. "I promise you. Your stories are just waiting for you to walk them out." I know this from experience. When I was writing my crime novel *The Dark Room,* I went for long daily walks. While I was admiring the first desert spring flowers, I was also concocting murder and mayhem. The more I wrote, the more I needed to walk. As I invented a dark and grisly world, I needed the stability and calm that walking gave me.

Walking yields us a sense of connection. We walk alone and yet we find ourselves a part of a larger world. "Walking makes me feel I am a part of the city," Denise reports of her daily walks in Manhattan. "Faces are often friendly, even in crowds. I like the sense that I am one among many, that I am on my rounds as others are on theirs."

For many city dwellers, a habit of walking yields them their first sense of the city as a friendly environment. "Before I started walking, the city seemed overwhelming to me," reports Jane, now an avid walker. "I overate to block my feelings of intimidation. Once I began walking, I began to see the city on a much smaller scale, neighborhood by neighborhood. Instead of a large and intimidating metropolis, I realized I lived in a world of interconnected neighborhoods. I also discovered many tiny markets containing fresh and wholesome foods. That inspired me to start cooking again, and as soon as I did, I began to feel more as if my home was really a home. As I got more comfortable in my own skin, my weight began to slowly slip away. I tucked the scale under the living room couch, where it has lived out its days."

When I lived in the country, my daily walks were also walks through a neighborhood of sorts. I learned: here is where the little water snakes live; here is where the coyotes dwell; here is the home of the rabbits and there the quail. I began to expect encounters with these creatures, to greet them the way a New Yorker might sight a neighbor.

"I've got coyotes in my far field," says Georgia, a painter who lives in the hill country of Wisconsin. "I've got bunnies in my garden. In the woods by the river trail, I often spot deer. If I'm lucky, I see a fox—not to mention all of the birds. When I hike as far as the wetlands, I see red-winged blackbirds, Canada geese, mallards, and an occasional heron." For Georgia, the fauna are her daily walking companions. "I think they know to expect me every afternoon between two and three. That's when I take a break from my painting."

For Georgia, walks are a sort of emotional sorbet, a palate-cleansing break between bouts at the easel. She has made walking a regular part of her daily schedule, and that is what is optimal for most of us. Some people find they like to walk right after their Morning Pages. They may walk to work—or part of the way to work, getting off the subway one or two stops early. Others walk at night, stretching their legs to unkink the stresses of the day. It matters less when you walk than that you walk. A daily walk is best. Such walks speed up your metabolism and allow you to burn calories with greater efficiency.

My daily walks fall midafternoon. Like Georgia, I use them to clear my palate, switching over from my work on music to my work on writing. Walking out of doors, I enjoy an image flow—there's a squirrel, here's a pinecone—and that image flow helps me to fill the creative pond. Back at home, when I fish for ideas, I find them.

When I cannot walk outside, I walk uphill on a treadmill, and as I do, I may cue up music or read from my favorite prayer book, *Creative Ideas* by Ernest Holmes. Like the sights of the natural world, the music and the prayers create a positive inflow. As I walk, my mood elevates, as does my perspective.

According to my doctor, Christopher Barley, himself a tall and lanky man with a metabolism a bird would envy, a brisk twenty-minute daily walk is enough. "You don't need to walk far or uphill," he says, "but you do need to walk daily. A daily walk can make for some astonishingly good results medically." Such results include lower cholesterol and weight. In my first month of daily walking, I lost nine pounds.

Walking, creative ideas will come to you. Walking, your appetite for bingeing will diminish. Next time you feel a Snack Attack, try taking a walk and record the results.

TASK

Walk Your Talk

Slip into your walking shoes. Lace them up. Comfortable? Good. Set out now for a twenty-minute walk. If you tell yourself you have no time, remember that walks make time. While walking, you get clear on your day's priorities. You move into the remainder of your day with a lighter heart. After your walk, you may wish to write down the insights, inspirations, and intuitions that came to you.

The Fourth Tool:
The Four Questions

The Snack Attack is a cunning enemy. It catches us off guard when our defenses are down. Let us say that we have put in a solid day of healthful eating. The Snack Attack will ambush us at bedtime. It will praise us for our virtue and tell us that "just a little bit" of something sinful won't hurt. But a little bit of something sinful does hurt—and the little bit often leads to just a little bit more.

My personal downfall is homemade cherry cake, a staple in my house since I live with an expert baker. Most mornings I wake to the scent of a freshly baked something. This morning, for example, it was a chocolate pistachio cake. Yesterday it was hazelnut brownies. I am adroit at facing down these delectable enemies. Chocolate, after all, is chocolate, the devil's food, and I know better than to indulge. Cherry cake, on the other hand, masquerades as something so light and innocent that surely a slice couldn't hurt. But a slice does hurt—one slice leads to another—and so I reach into my tool kit for a series of four questions aimed at defusing the dietary bombshell.

"Am I hungry?" runs question number one. I have discovered that very often, the answer to that question is no. I am not hungry, but I am bored or frustrated and the slice of cake poses as a culinary adventure. Faced with a blank page, I may turn to the refrigerator instead. By asking "Am I hungry?" there's a chance I may derail the dietary train wreck before it happens. But if I am hungry, I move on to question number two.

"Is this what I want to eat?" asks question number two. This is another question designed to stop a Snack Attack in its tracks. Anthony tells the story of craving a cheeseburger until he asked himself this question and discovered that no, he did not want all of the calories, all of the grease and carbs. "What I ended up eating was a fresh sweet peach," he says. "I discovered that because it's sweet, fruit often kills a Snack Attack with kindness."

"Is this what I want to eat now?" asks question number three. Many dieters report that Snack Attacks come at them late at night. "It was my bogeyman, the midnight Snack Attack guaranteed to go straight to my hips," recalls Margie. "I believed Oprah when she said I shouldn't eat late at night, but shouldn't didn't mean wouldn't. Two nights out of three, I gave in to temptation, and that temptation showed up on the next morning's scale. The truth is," continues Margie, "I often don't want a fattening something in the middle of the night. I tell myself I can always have it the next day."

Question number four holds the key to freedom for someone like Margie. "Is there something that I can eat instead?" asks this question, and it opens the door for smart substitutions. Often the solution is to stock your refrigerator with foods that are legal at any hour. Far better to have a late night diet Jell-O or pudding than a midnight Häagen-Dazs binge. A plum instead of Mallomars.

Above all else, overeaters eat—but with the help of the four questions they eat more sensibly.

"I found that with the regular use of the four questions, I channeled my eating along much healthier lines," confides Jeanette. "When I was hit by a Snack Attack, I would ask myself the questions. Very often I was able to make a healthy substitution if not avoid snacking altogether. Using the questions, I lost ten pounds that had stayed stubbornly stuck."

"What I liked about the questions were their realism," says Lucy. "They squarely faced the fact that I probably was going to eat something, and they helped me to make that something that would do the least damage. I cannot tell you the number of times I passed up cookies for a bowl of butterless popcorn."

"The questions taught me the value of fruit," laughs Anthony, a tall and handsome lawyer who had routinely carried an extra forty pounds. "I retrained my sweet tooth to be satisfied with natural sugar. I would crave something sweet and find that I could eat a bowl of strawberries with Splenda or a sliced peach." In the first month that he worked with the questions, Anthony took off nine pounds, but he found his psychology shifted as much as his physique. "Instead of deprivation and resentment, my usual dieting companions, I felt a growing sense of competency. I realized that I was actually learning a new lifestyle with healthy eating habits."

Carlos, who worked as a waiter serving delectable and fattening foods on a cruise ship, found that it helped him to carry the questions written out in his pocket. "Chef was always putting out 'treats' for the staff. I found that by using the questions I could turn the fattening treats down. Very often I wasn't hungry. If I was hungry, I very often didn't really want to eat what was being offered."

Using the questions defensively, Carlos lost inches and pounds in the first month. "I am really starting to look different," he exulted to me. "I am starting to think of myself as good-looking, not just chubby. And maybe it's because I'm cuter or maybe it's because my attitude has improved—so have my tips!"

An improved attitude, greater optimism, more energy—these are the rewards of working regularly with the four questions. As easy as a game, the ritual of asking the four questions gently but thoroughly awakens our awareness of exactly when we are eating and what. Those questions again:

1. Am I hungry?
2. Is this what I feel like eating?
3. Is this what I feel like eating now?
4. Is there something else that I could eat instead?

TASK

Asking the Four Questions

Take pen in hand. Ask yourself, "What is my attitude toward using the four questions?" Do you have a favorite? Write about it in detail. Do you have one that often pays off? Is there one you tend to skip? Has question number four helped you to alter the contents of your refrigerator?

The Fifth Tool:
Culinary Artist Dates

Most of us dread dieting, associating it with hardship and deprivation. But what if healthful eating was actually fun? What if your diet involved culinary adventures rather than sheer abstinence? The Writing Diet proposes that you take a festive, creative culinary outing once a week. Grounded in creativity theory, the Culinary Artist Date is a variation on a tried-and-true recovery tool, the Artist Date, which is a weekly solo expedition aimed at gently expanding your comfort zone. As the name suggests, this is a tool aimed at self-romancing. On these dates you become intimate with yourself. An Artist Date is sacred time. Think pleasure, not duty. Choose an outing that enchants you. In planning and executing your Culinary Artist Date, expect to encounter a certain amount of resistance. Despite its seeming frivolity, this is a serious tool for self-discovery. A Culinary Artist Date might involve dining out. It might entail a trip to Williams-Sonoma, a fine cookware store. You might take a cooking lesson or go to a farmers' market.

"Call me a classicist," says Raina. "Once a week I crave a really good cheeseburger. I've been all over New York comparing and contrasting what's offered. My favorite is a guacamole burger, medium rare, charbroiled. I eat it without the bun, and with a side salad instead of french fries. I find I satisfy my craving for something naughty while still staying within the guidelines for healthful eating."

Not all of us subscribe to Raina's taste in Americana—not when there is sushi to be had, not when we can get good Chinese or Ethiopian food, not when we live close to Little Italy and not far from Koreatown.

"I had a terrible fear of dining out alone," relates Charlotte. "I had to screw my courage to the sticking post the first time I tried this adventure. Surely, I thought, everyone will notice that I'm alone. Everyone will think I'm weird. Everyone will think I'm a loser. To my delight, no one seemed to think any such thing. Looking around the restaurant, I wasn't the only solo diner. This gave me courage. I had brought a book with me so that I could tune out my environment, but I found I wanted to tune in instead. I was interested by the waiters. I was interested by the other diners. Dining out solo did seem like an adventure. I couldn't wait to try it again."

Many of us, like Charlotte, have learned to love our Culinary Artist Dates. We have learned to plan ahead, anticipating the meal we will have and the time we will spend in our own good company.

"Dining out alone became one of the high points of my week," says Susan. "It was a special adventure for me, and one that I learned to plot out ahead of time. I began collecting menus on my walks. Safe at home, I would pore over them, selecting that week's expedition. Should it be Thai? What about Mexican? Maybe Japanese? Or my favorite fallback, Chinese?"

Like Susan, many of us began collecting menus on our walks. Ethnic food doesn't necessarily mean fattening food. At a Chinese restaurant, ask for your meat and vegetables steamed with sauce on the side for dipping. Indian food? All that buttered bread? Try tandoori chicken instead. Deli food loomed as perhaps the most dangerous, but we found we could eat the fillings of deli sandwiches and avoid the bread. (Good deli pickles are practically calorie free!) Delis also make many salads and savory, nonfattening soups.

"I'm not Jewish," explains Emily, "but I've discovered that I love good Jewish food. Week after week I venture out to delis. I eat pastrami sandwiches. I eat tongue. I eat chopped chicken liver. I eat matzo ball soup. What I don't eat is the New York–style cheesecake. Instead, I go home to my special dessert of whipped ricotta and frozen fruit."

Food itself is not the enemy. Our use and abuse of food is the issue. Learning to dine out well and carefully is a social skill that stands us in good stead. It takes energy to say no when we are tempted by the bread basket—better to think of it as saying yes to something else. This is why studying the menu ahead of time can be a great asset. Often there are healthful appetizers and salads that are all too easily overlooked.

"I live in Manhattan," says Glenda. "It's a mecca for dining out. I started with my own neighborhood, but as I got braver, I tried out Chinatown, Little Italy, Koreatown, Japantown, and Little Brazil. I discovered I had a real taste for exotic cuisine. I added to my own supply of spices for the nights I cooked in."

Many of us discover that our Culinary Artist Dates give us a sense of well-being and adventure. We aren't "trapped" on a diet. Instead, we are learning a new and expansive lifestyle.

"I can't tell you how hard it was taking myself out alone," confesses Victoria, a thirty-something single. "I thought everyone would stare at me. Instead, I found I was treated with courtesy and respect. It was as if everyone wanted me to have a particularly nice time, and I did." Victoria, an Italian-American, found herself gravitating toward Little Italy and the cuisine of her ancestors. "It wasn't all pasta. There was veal, fish, antipasto. I found I could eat lean and clean, although the great Italian bread was always tempting. I let myself have a slice if I skipped the tartufo for dessert."

Many of us find that dining out alone pays off in unexpected social dividends. We find ourselves able to be graceful—and to know that we are graceful. Able to decline rich foods we do not want, we become skilled at finding "legal" delicacies.

"I found I could channel my appetite along healthy lines," says Regina. "I'd order some lean protein and several sides of vegetables. Sometimes I would make a fine meal on appetizers alone. With no one else to watch over what I ate, I found myself choosing wisely and well—just a little eccentrically."

Many of us find that our Culinary Artist Dates give us permission to explore and "own" our own appetites. There is no one sitting across from us to question our choices. We're able to select exactly what strikes our fancy and fits our pocketbook. Dining out is not so expensive, especially if you skip dessert and cappuccinos.

"I'm crazy about bacon, lettuce, and tomato sandwiches," says Stacy. "I find them emotionally satisfying. And if I'm careful with my food for the rest of the day, I can 'afford' them."

Whether we opt for a modest BLT or a more sumptuous feast, treating ourselves to dinner out is a part of treating ourselves well.

TASK

Planning Your Date

Find a comfortable chair. Curl up with your journal and ask yourself the following question: What would I love eating? The answer may surprise you. You may crave a simple cheeseburger, a calzone, or exotic Ethiopian fare. Is it a specific spice you are craving? Is there a taste you long to taste? What would constitute a perfect meal for you? Plan it on the page.

The Sixth Tool:
HALT

Newcomers to alcohol abstinence are advised in 12-step parlance to observe the acronym HALT. As they work to establish abstinence, they are repeatedly told, "Don't get too Hungry, Angry, Lonely, or Tired." Those four conditions render the recovering alcoholic vulnerable to picking up a drink. In trying to establish dietary sobriety, it is also advisable to observe HALT. If we get too hungry, too angry, too lonely, or too tired, we are vulnerable to overeating.

"I needed to learn to eat regular meals. When I skipped a meal, I got too hungry and then I binged," says Janet, a once-plump filmmaker who has chiseled off pounds. "It was the 'H' in HALT that always sabotaged me. I kept going long after I was burned out. Then I used food to fuel my overwork."

"I got a lot of mileage out of being 'nice,'" says Benjamin, a portly composer. "Whenever I felt angry, I ate to stuff my feelings. I never expressed how I really felt; instead, I had another serving of cheesecake or macaroni and cheese. I used comfort foods to console myself. When I began using a journal, I began to feel my feelings without acting on them. I found I could calmly and maturely express my anger. I may not be quite as 'nice' anymore, but I am a hell of a lot thinner."

"That makes me very angry," we might write instead of eating the last piece of cheesecake. The cake is a sedative that dulls our emotions, while anger is a spark that can be used as creative fuel. Entire books, plays, and operas have been written out of anger. The creative arena is the best possible arena in which to express anger. Anger gave us Picasso's *Guernica*. Anger gave us Pasternak's *Doctor Zhivago*. Properly channeled, anger is a lodestone for creative endeavors. So why does it have such a bad reputation?

Most of us are uncomfortable with our anger. We have been taught that it is "bad," perhaps "unspiritual." We forget that Christ himself lost his temper with the money changers in the temple. He felt his anger and it galvanized him to action. He acted on it correctly. We can do the same thing. We can take our anger to the page and write (right) our emotions. We write to tell ourselves the truth—and the truth may be that we are angry. HA!

Sara, a proud and successful woman, suffered an unhappy marriage to a jealous and competitive man. When he left her for a younger woman, she spiraled into depression. She began to stuff her uncomfortable feelings with nightly ice cream binges. The pounds crept on. When I met her, she was pudgy and miserable. She was also blocked in her work as a painter. I suggested that she write instead of binge—and that she allow herself to write about her ex-husband just as bitterly and angrily as she felt. "Don't worry about writing well," I told her. "Write badly. Write anything at all." Dubious at first, Sara tried writing. Her very first poem shot onto the page:

This little poem goes out to my ex.
I think I ought to use a hex.
He was jealous of me and my art.
Whatever I made, he tore apart.
He felt envy of all that I made.
He could have tried but he was afraid . . .
He got his laughs tearing me down
But I was the winner, he was the clown.

Sara called me up thrilled and excited. Writing instead of bingeing was like taking truth serum, she reported. She suddenly saw things clearly. The ice cream was forgotten in the excitement of the naughty fun that she was having. Did I realize, she wondered, that her ex-husband was passive-aggressive? She was better off without him. At my suggestion Sara established a writing practice: Morning Pages first thing in the day, quick little poems in her journal for whenever she felt a Snack Attack coming on.

"I feel like Picasso," she reported excitedly after a few days. "I'm making art out of anything and everything." As Sara expressed the feelings she had been stuffing with food, she soon stopped overeating. In fact, I had to remind her to eat, she got so caught up in her creative projects. "Creativity versus negativity" became her banner. She posted her logo on a little sign by her computer. When feelings, particularly those of anger, struck, she would strike the keys. A page at a time, she put much-needed distance and perspective between her and her ex-husband. She began making art "at" him and found that she just loved making art for its own sweet sake. The extra pounds began to come off.

"I was Miss Lonelyhearts," recalls Candace, who spent long,

lonely evenings with the TV for company and Cinnabons or buttered popcorn for consolation. "I watched a lot of romantic comedies, but my weight was no laughing matter. When I started practicing HALT, I saw that 'lonely' was my Achilles' heel. I made a pact with a friend that I would phone her before I ate anything. The calls attacked my loneliness directly. The buttered popcorn became a thing of the past."

"We all know that food is fuel," asserts Judith, a type-A personality who believed that if work was good, overwork was even better. "I always brought work home from the office, and when I would start to drag, I would eat to jack myself up. My favorite combo was caffeine and sugar. I could go through a whole package of Oreos, all the while feeling virtuous because I was working." For Judith, "tired" was the part of HALT that rendered her vulnerable to bingeing.

Nestor, a car salesman, has a useful analogy. "I think of HALT as being like the message lights on the dashboard. Whenever one of the letters flickers on, I have to pay attention and get myself proper maintenance."

"Proper maintenance" may mean a healthy snack, a session writing out feelings in our journal, a visit with a friend, or an evening of early-to-bed. When we learn, like Nestor, to think of our body as a delicate mechanism requiring care, we start to be alert to the kind of care required.

"I've come to think of myself as an ecosystem," reports Kathleen, a marine biologist. "I have to monitor myself for HALT the same way I monitor a fish tank so that it doesn't get too alkaline. It's all a matter of balance. I need to be alert to conditions."

For many of us, being alert to conditions is a matter of heightened consciousness. We are accustomed to abusing ourselves. We routinely allow ourselves to become too hungry, too angry, too lonely, or too tired. Very often we tell ourselves that such conditions are normal. This is an unconscious rationalization: "You'd eat, too, if you had my miserable life."

Life becomes a lot less miserable the instant we start practicing HALT. When we begin to treat ourselves like precious objects, we begin to grow strong. As we grow strong, our weakness for overeating diminishes.

TASK

How do you do at HALT?

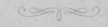

Take pen in hand. Set aside a half hour. This is a time for honest self-scrutiny. Describe your relationship to each of the warning words in HALT. Do you get too hungry? Too angry? Too lonely? Too tired? Are any—or all—triggers for you? What can you do to alter this fact? For example, do you need to learn the art of the catnap? The phone call? The preemptive prayer? Often you can "design" a new behavior on the page, then put it into practice in your life. You may want to check in with your Body Buddy (see next essay) to see if there's a HALT signal that you have missed. Your Body Buddy may have noticed a pattern that you have missed.

The Seventh Tool:
The Body Buddy

Y ou're beautiful just the way you are," we are often told. Burdened by overweight, however, we do not *feel* beautiful. We may feel quite the opposite. As we begin the regimen of the Writing Diet, our emotions may be turbulent, and our self-image may fluctuate terribly. Objectively we need to lose "some" weight. Subjectively that "sum" may be too much for us to handle—at least alone. What we need is an ally, someone to cheer us on, someone to believe in us and our objectives. That someone might best be called a Body Buddy.

What is a Body Buddy? It is an objective person with whom you can be completely candid. This means the person must be selected with care. You do not want an enabler, someone who tells you you don't need to lose weight, that your inner beauty shines forth. Nor do you need a punitive "keeper," someone who treats each mouthful you consume as a crime. You are looking for a person who is balanced, kind, and yet objective. Ideally you will check in with this person daily.

Working with your journal, you have an accurate log of each

day's eating. It is wise to share this log daily. It helps you to acknowledge your gains and your slips. This is where the Body Buddy proves invaluable.

"You were doing pretty well until happy hour," your Body Buddy might note. "What happened then?"

"I got an upsetting business call when it was too late to do anything about it," you may remember. Frustrated and frightened, you turned to food.

"At least you didn't binge the entire rest of the day," your Body Buddy may add encouragingly.

"No, it was just those three handfuls of nuts. Maybe they're a trigger food for me?"

"Maybe they are. Why don't you try stocking up on a different form of protein?"

The Body Buddy loves us as we are, with all our faults and failings, and yet agrees with our goal of weight loss. It is often difficult at first to be candid with this chosen confidant. We are afraid to share the late-night eating binge. We worry about judgment. We dread condemnation. What we meet with instead is objectivity.

"So you binged last night. How are you doing so far today?"

"Pretty well, I guess."

"Well, then, good. Let's focus on today."

With the help of our Body Buddy, we stay on track. We are held accountable for our actions. Often, our Body Buddy will see things that we don't, hidden stresses that repeatedly trigger us to overeat. The Body Buddy may also devise strategies that serve to curb our appetites—strategies like exercise.

"Did you get on the treadmill today?" a Body Buddy might ask.

"Why, yes, I did."

"Well, good, then. I've noticed that when you exercise you tend to not overeat. I actually think exercise curbs your appetite. Do you agree?"

Many times a Body Buddy will raise issues of self-care that we have been neglecting. A Body Buddy might ask, "Have you cleaned out your refrigerator and gotten rid of your trigger foods?" A Body Buddy might ask, "Are you drinking your full sixty-four ounces of water a day?"

Sometimes your Body Buddy is a fellow overeater. In such cases, the check-ins are often reciprocal. This breeds compassion and empathy. Listening to someone else's struggles, we often feel a burst of sympathy for our own.

"Be kind to yourself," we might caution our Body Buddy.

"And what about you?" our Body Buddy might counter.

Working at its best, the Body Buddy constitutes a system of checks and balances. We check in on our day and we balance our eating and exercise for successful weight loss. Many people report that it is in contact with their Body Buddy that they experience a spiritual helping hand in their weight-loss program.

"Christ said, 'Wherever two or more are gathered together, there I am in the midst,' " says Joyce. "Talking with my Body Buddy, I often experience a sense of forgiveness and grace. I am able to feel compassion for relapses and hope for a better future."

While many of us succeed in establishing a bond with our very first choice of Body Buddy, others of us find we must try, try again.

"My first choice in a Body Buddy was a real Nazi," laughs Joanna. "I picked someone very rigid, who was 'perfect' on her food plan. She expected the same perfection from me, and was very shaming whenever I fell off the wagon. After six months I found myself feeling bludgeoned and bullied. There was no focus on how well I was doing, only on my slip-ups. I want someone more positive, I decided. That's when I met Claire. In 12-step terms, she 'had what I wanted.' "

When Joanna met Claire, she recognized the health of Claire's attitudes toward food and her body. Claire was trim and fit and attractive. Neither fat nor skinny, she carried her weight easily, moving with zest and enthusiasm. Her clothes fit easily, neither too tight nor too baggy. She didn't hide her body, but she didn't flaunt it either. She was a graceful woman.

"The first thing that impressed me about Claire was her emphasis on the positive. She gave me a great deal of reinforcement for what I did right. When I would slip up on a day's eating, her emphasis was always to get me straight back on track rather than to wallow in regret. From Claire I learned that I could start my day over again anytime. I didn't need to see a binge through to the bitter end. I could interrupt it. 'Call me,' Claire said. 'Call me *before* you binge.' It took me a while to do that, but when I did, I found I was able to stop a binge in its tracks. My binges were due to loneliness, to the feeling it was me against the world. Claire put an end to my self-destructive solitude."

TASK

Selecting a Body Buddy

Take pen in hand. On the page, as specifically as possible, describe what you would hope to find in a Body Buddy. What characteristics do you feel you need? What mixture of kindness, humor, compassion, and accountability is right for you? Some people believe that they need tough love, and indeed, it may be right for them. Others yearn for a more lenient approach, and that can work also. Once you have outlined for yourself what it is you are seeking, ask yourself the next question: Is there anyone in my acquaintance who fills the bill? You may sense immediately the perfect partner for you. If you do, fine. Place a phone call, explain what you're up to, and forge a partnership for yourself. Some of us find no immediate partner springs to mind. This requires prayer, patience, and footwork. Sometimes a partner steps forward from the most unexpected quarters. Marjorie forged a Body Buddy bond with a younger gay man whom she met through her night school class. Despite the difference in their sexes and a thirty-year gap in their ages, they were very compatible, sharing a wry sense of humor and a determination to become more fit. Since both of them were computer geeks, they found it natural to do their check-ins by e-mail. They soon enjoyed a lively correspondence.

In choosing a Body Buddy, take care to pick someone who is emotionally available, whether by phone, in person, or by e-mail. Physical proximity is less important than emotional availability. Choose someone whom you like as well as admire. Remember that the relationship can be intimate, and it is important to pick someone you can trust.

Part Two

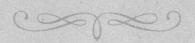

SITUATIONS

and

SOLUTIONS

What Is Sensible
Eating Anyhow?

We know more about what sensible eating is not than about what it is. We know, for example, that sensible eating does not involve two heavily laden slices of pizza and an outsize Coke. We know that it's a no to devour half a dozen chocolate chip cookies no matter how healthy the glass of milk may be with which we wash them all down. We know that fried chicken and biscuits are delicious but highly caloric. We know that half of a Sara Lee cake will show up as inches on our hips.

Some of us also know what works for us. We know that Weight Watchers works for us or that South Beach works for us. Others of us do not know, and there are few more painful places to be than not knowing how to begin. I am not a nutritionist, but I have worked with a nutritionist, Sara Ryba, an esteemed expert in the field of weight control. She believes in a plan she calls Clean Eating. This has worked for me, and it may provide you with a useful jumping-off place.

What is Clean Eating? It certainly sounds good and, I am happy to report, it tastes good as well. At its best, Clean Eating is sensible eating, nothing too radical, nothing too strict. You eat lean when you eat moderately. You do not weigh or measure food, but you do need to be conscious of portion sizes. You stop bingeing on the deadly whites—sugar, flour, starches. You start drinking water, lots and lots of water—at least eight eight-ounce glasses per day. You eat three meals a day and two small snacks, all modest in calories but not punitively so. Clean food is food as close to its natural state as possible. (It's useful to remember that overprocessed adds to overweight.) That means crisp fresh vegetables and fruits, low-fat dairy products, lean proteins, and whole grains. If you eat clean ninety percent of the time, you are eating for weight loss and optimal health.

A DAY IN THE LIFE

Breakfast: coffee or tea with milk, ½ cup yogurt or ricotta with 1 cup sliced berries—or a fruit smoothie with yogurt, berries, and a little Splenda

Snack: 10 almonds or two cheese sticks, a low-cal granola bar, or those old standby celery sticks

Lunch: 4 ounces lean protein with 2 cups salad greens (use a low-sugar, olive oil–based dressing). This might be a salad Niçoise. Use 4 ounces tuna packed in water, two cups salad greens, ½ sliced bell pepper, ¼ cup sliced red onion, one medium tomato cut into wedges, and two tablespoons low-fat vinaigrette.

Snack: 1 Granny Smith apple with 1 ounce hard cheese, a wedge of Laughing Cow cheese, or a cup of vegetable soup

Dinner: 4 ounces lean protein—perhaps grilled chicken or salmon—with 3 cups cooked vegetables sautéed in olive oil and ½ cup brown rice

Dessert: decaf cappuccino with skim milk and Splenda, sugar-free Jell-O, or ricotta whipped with fruit, a South Beach favorite

Eating clean takes a bit of fine-tuning. Some bodies can metabolize more grains or dairy than others. As a rule, the more muscle mass you have, the more you can eat. Metabolism is a matter of genetics and luck, but the one way you can change your metabolism is through exercise. Athletes can get away with eating an enviable amount of food, but they also work hard to work it off. Most of us need to eat just a little less and exercise just a little more to gradually take off pounds.

As a basic rule, if you are still hungry, you need more food. If you are full, it's time to stop. If you are not sure, then you need to write about it. Many of us experience the phenomenon of false hunger, and we must train ourselves to discern the real thing. This is where the four questions come in handy. This is where the journal proves its value. Remember, we are trying to write our way right-size.

TASK

What's "Write" Eating?

How close do you come to the ideal of Clean Eating? In a nutshell, it's low carbs, low fats, no refined sugar, and careful portion control. Three meals a day and two healthy snacks should be enough to keep you from feeling deprived. It's a plan that works for many people, but it may not be the one you choose. If you are reading this book, the odds are excellent that you are a veteran dieter. Let's take a look at what experience has taught you.

Do you know what plan works for you? You may have dropped out of an eating plan that did work when you worked it. With the help of the Writing Diet's tool kit, you may be able to return to a plan that was a known winner. Your written insights may show you just how and why you sabotaged yourself. You may well be able to set such sabotage aside. Alternatively, you may feel that the plan you tried to work was wrong for you. For example, Weight Watchers acknowledges two different temperaments by giving members the choice between counting points or eating only from "core" foods. A point person doesn't do well on core and vice versa. You do know yourself well enough to know what's up your alley and what seems out of the question for your personality.

Pen in hand, ask yourself what has been your experience in the past with eating plans. Without judging yourself, try to judge how different plans work for you. Is there a food or food group you simply cannot give up despite its evident toxicity? You may need a special detox period to get this substance under your control. It can be done.

Do you have an idea of your own downfalls in regard to Clean Eating? Is it portion control? Is it wrong foods? Write about all of this. This is an exploratory exercise to see how much you already know about yourself and your eating patterns. It's more than you suspect. For greater objectivity, try writing about yourself in the third person: "She experienced great success with Atkins, but her cholesterol zoomed. . . ." "She did well on Weight Watchers until she began to seriously weight-train. Then she needed more than the allotted points."

Your thumbnail sketch of yourself as a dieter should give you sufficient data to choose a food plan that works for you. Remember that the tools of the Writing Diet will work in combination with any food plan you choose. Often the shift in consciousness that comes from use of the tools is sufficient to cause weight loss even without a formal food plan in place. As you become more sensitive to yourself, your eating habits naturally improve. You may wish to share your findings from this tool with your Body Buddy.

Am I hungry
Is "this" what's feel
"this" what I feel
like eating?
Is. This what I feel
like eating now?
Is there something I
could eat instead?

The Snack Attack

I think of Snack Attacks as being a lot like B movies: everything is going along fine, when suddenly, from out of the shadows, IT appears. The "it" in a Snack Attack is the sinister little voice that suggests that it won't "really" hurt if you have "just a little." But a little of what? Ice cream? Taco chips? Homemade brownies? Asked to name our poison, most of us can tell you what we really shouldn't have in the house. For me, it's cherry cake. For my sister, it's nuts.

"I told myself nuts were healthy," says Claire. "And maybe a few nuts are healthy, but I never stopped at a few. I could eat handfuls of almonds, peanuts, or cashews. Nuts may be packed with healthy nutrients, but they're also packed with calories. I finally told myself, 'Nuts to nuts!'"

"Ice cream is good for you," Monty told himself. "It's dairy more than sugar." Every night he would tell himself one scoop was OK with the evening news. "But the news kept getting worse and the scoops kept getting bigger." As did Monty's waist.

Natalie, a vegetarian, believed wholeheartedly that her home-made guacamole and chips were a healthful snack. She prided herself on not eating processed foods, and she used only blue corn chips for her treat. She was surprised, given her "virtuous" eating, that she put on two full dress sizes. "I guess I'm a little bit of a grazer," she admitted.

Snack Attacks tell us that they are harmless. They play into our rationalizations: "You got on the bike today; you can afford some potato chips." Snack Attacks come when we are bored or when we have a difficult emotion we don't really want to face. We snack when we are hungry, angry, lonely, or tired, but we also snack when we are sad, joyful, excited—anytime when an emotion catches us off guard.

Michael snacked alone, late at night. After a day full of people and virtue, he would stop off for a triple cheeseburger on his way home. "Each night, it was like a mugging. The Snack Attack always caught me by surprise. The next day I'd feel hungover, exactly as if I had binged on alcohol."

For some of us, alcohol is the binge. "I'd save my Weight Watchers points so that I could have a nightcap," says Mandy. "Then I'd have two. I simply couldn't let a day go past without a couple of drinks."

What do we do when faced with a Snack Attack? Instead of acting out, we can take a new, healthy action. We can turn to the four questions, asking, "Am I hungry? Is this what I want to eat? Is this what I want to eat now? Is there something else that I could eat instead?" We can turn to our journal, asking ourselves, "What am I not expressing?" We can also turn to our

Higher Power, however we conceptualize it. We can pray, "Please help me now."

Agatha, a young composer, found that she often ate to avoid her next creative action. She found that when she prayed, she was often directed to her next right step. "I'd have a song to orchestrate and instead I would start fantasizing about peanut butter cookies. If I ate the cookies, I would forget all about the song. If I prayed, I would forget about the cookies. I would feel empowered about the song and about food. When my focus is on what it's supposed to be on—writing music—food falls into place. I am not preoccupied with it."

"Food was what I did instead of life," claims Fred, a recovering overeater. "I not only stuffed my feelings, I stuffed my actions. Let's say I had something pressing to do, like make a difficult phone call. I would eat something first, but it would end up being that I would eat something instead. After a Big Mac, the phone call just didn't seem to matter as much."

Glenda, a novelist, claims that her free-flowing prose is a result of getting sober about food. "I had to learn to write instead of eat," she says. "I found that if I binged, I not only stuffed my own feelings, I stuffed my characters' feelings as well."

Make no mistake, Snack Attacks are lethal. They add not only to our physical weight but to our psychic weight as well. Instead of facing the difficult conversation we need to have with our spouse, we turn to the refrigerator for understanding. As the pounds pile up, so do the resentments. We leave too many things unsaid, even when our lover asks us the telltale question "What's eating you?"

Snack Attacks are a bar to intimacy—and not just with our mates. Mothers report that they suffer Snack Attacks just when their children come home from school needing to make emotional contact and process the day's events. "I would suddenly be starving," relates Carrie. "I would make peanut butter and jelly for the kids and some for me."

For those of us who drink, happy hour is often a Snack Attack in liquid form.

"My husband and I would share a couple of cocktails and news of the day," recalls Jane. "It was our nightly ritual to get just a little sloshed as we debriefed."

Stoned from a sugar high, sloshed from a stiff cocktail, the Snack Attack leaves us emotionally impaired. Life happens in a haze. We disconnect from ourselves and then from others.

For Maggie, Snack Attacks came every night at bedtime. "When my husband felt like making love, I felt like eating pizza," she confesses. "After a pizza, who needs sex?"

I suggested to Maggie that she might want to try working with the four questions. Question number one was all that it took to shock her into clarity. She discovered she wasn't hungry at all— just anxious about her sexual performance. "I'd been putting weight on ever since the birth of our second child. When I gave up pizza and late-night snacks, I found I once more had an appetite for sex. My husband was thrilled."

For many overeaters, the Snack Attack is a substitute for sex. For all too many of us, food is love, even sexual love. Karl, a good-looking gay man, packed on a full fifty pounds and entered, no co-incidence, a prolonged period of celibacy. "Food was my partner,"

Karl says now. "I used food to meet my needs for physical satis-faction and comfort. I used food to meet my needs for intimacy. Every night I'd make a big bowl of buttered popcorn or buy a bag of taco chips. I'd watch a movie and talk to the screen."

Karl's entry to recovery was bumpy. Some days he would do his Morning Pages and work with his questions; other days he would binge. "I kept sabotaging myself," he says. "I just wasn't ready to face my own turbulent emotions. I really wanted a lov-ing, committed partner and I believed I would never get one."

After several months of skidding back and forth, Karl com-mitted to being more conscious about his food and everything else in his life. A day at a time, a sentence at a time, he came to clar-ity, and as he did so, the weight began to melt away. "I am still too chubby," he said in the ad he placed with an Internet dating serv-ice. His candor won him the attention of an "interested party" who soon would evolve into his partner and mate.

For many of us, like Karl, it takes some time to commit. While we can see how creative recovery could work in principle, we would still rather binge than face ourselves on the page. Until we are fully committed—and committed to vigilance—Snack Attacks are often dietary U-turns. We do well "until."

"I had a habit of being conscious only about fifty percent of the time," says Jeannie, who routinely found herself sabotaged by Snack Attacks. "Eventually, through the use of Morning Pages, my journal, and the four questions, I became more alert. Now a Snack Attack seldom catches me by surprise."

TASK

Attacking the Snack Attack

Take pen in hand. Describe a typical Snack Attack for you. When does it occur? Is there a recurring pattern? Is there a trigger emotion? How do you rationalize a Snack Attack? What do you do to make up for it once the attack is over? Do you purge? Do you overexercise? Do you starve yourself, denying yourself the "luxury" of a regular meal? Again, share your findings with your Body Buddy.

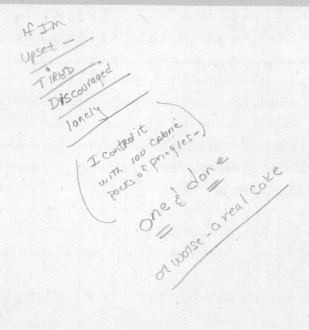

If I'm
upset -
TIRED
Discouraged
lonely

I control it
with 100 calorie
pacts of pringles -

One & done

or worse - a real coke

The First Bite:
Trigger Foods

The Writing Diet makes us conscious of our behaviors generally and our behaviors around food particularly. Many of us notice that we have a deep-seated denial when it comes to dealing with Snack Attacks. "What will one little bite hurt?" we say to ourselves. We are unwilling or unable to face the fact that it is the first bite that leads to the binge. Recovering alcoholics are taught that it is the first drink that leads to a drunk. They do not need to worry about the second drink or the seventh drink. They need only avoid the first one and all else will be safe and sane. The same can be said with overeating. Certain foods are like drinks for us. They lead to binge behavior. We simply cannot eat them safely. These foods are our trigger foods.

"Anything white," Helen characterizes her trigger foods. "Sugar, refined flour, bread, pasta, potatoes."

"Anything salty," volunteers Bernice, who cannot safely take the first chip.

"For me it's fatty foods," says Eleanor. "It sounds awful, but I crave grease. Give me anything that's deep fried and I cannot stop eating it—french fries, fried calamari, southern fried chicken. . . . The first bite leads to the binge."

"I have learned I cannot have certain foods in the house," says Jackie. "The first butterscotch leads to the bag of butterscotch. The first spoonful of Nutella leads to devouring the entire jar."

"I think it's easier for an alcoholic," says Mark. "After all, an alcoholic can simply quit. An overeater still has to eat."

We do still have to eat, but what we eat, why we eat, and how we eat can all be made conscious. We can learn healthy eating behaviors and we can teach them to ourselves through writing. Morning Pages give us the big picture of our day. We see the stresses that may cause us to want to act out with food. Throughout the day, use of the journal helps us to dismantle each Snack Attack as it is upon us. The four questions lead us into healthier eating choices. We learn to name and avoid our trigger foods. Sometimes with the help of a quickly uttered prayer, we gain the strength to resist the first bite.

"For me, it was macaroni and cheese," says Sheila. "I called it my comfort food, but I wasn't very comfortable after bingeing on it."

"Home fries were my trigger food," recalls Arthur. "An omelet just looked naked to me without them. The first time I said, 'Hold the fries,' I thought I was going to die. Since then I've learned to ask for a side of something 'legal,' like spinach or lettuce and tomato. I no longer feel quite so deprived, and now I'll admit my weight to my partner. For over a year, it had been my deep, dark secret."

TASK

The Deep, Dark Secret

Most of us have secrets related to our overeating. Some of us have thrown food away—only to go into the trash and retrieve it. Others of us have binged, then purged, forcing ourselves to vomit up the food we have just gulped down. Take pen in hand and write out your worst secret related to food. Do you eat raw cookie dough? Do you binge on ice cream? Is a huge vat of buttered popcorn your addiction? Is it Froot Loops? Mars bars? DoveBars? Get the details onto the page. What did you do and how did it make you feel? Write it out. Share your discoveries with your Body Buddy.

Angela tells the story of her Nutella binge. "I began with a few spoonfuls. Then I said, 'I must throw this out.' I threw the Nutella in the kitchen trash and went into my room. A few minutes later I was back in the kitchen into the trash. 'I'd better throw this all the way out,' I thought. I took the trash out to the hall. A few minutes later, there I was out in the hall, eating the Nutella out of the trash. Nutella is one of the most addictive substances I know. I have to understand that if I am going to buy a jar of Nutella, I am going to eat the whole thing. I found that once I was willing to write this secret out and became willing to share it with other people, I found I wasn't the only one who had been struck by the Nutella curse."

Special Occasions

*I*n my house, growing up, Christmas began in October. That was when my mother began baking—and freezing—the special treats that signified the holiday. She made batches of fudge and divinity. She made sugar cookies and toffee bars. She made pecan balls and orange date-nut bread. Each day I would walk in the door from school and inhale the scent of a freshly baked delicacy wafting through the house.

My mother had special menus for all special occasions, not just Christmas. Take Thanksgiving, for example. There was Thanksgiving turkey with all the trimmings: corn meal and sage dressings, sweet potatoes, cheese-creamed onions, asparagus, two kinds of cranberry relish, crescent rolls. Easter, Halloween, New Year's, Fourth of July—each had its special dishes. Food signified "holiday" and "celebration." I grew up steeped in a rich culinary tradition. Now that I am grown, living in Manhattan instead of in the heartland, I find that food still signifies special occasions—but that the number and diversity of possible occasions has multiplied. I have friends who celebrate Hanukkah with latkes and fried doughnuts, friends who celebrate the feast of Beltane with roast pig. All of my friends and all of their occasions feature delicious signature foods.

"Food makes the holiday," states my friend Linda. "Food speaks of tradition, continuity, and family. And don't try to make any modern, low-fat latkes. Go for the real deal."

In other words, food is political and the act of not eating special foods is seen as treasonous. "Surely you can have a tiny bite!" offended family bakers urge. Often we have the first bite and many more bites after that. After all, we want to belong, and food signifies belonging.

"Firsts weren't enough. In my family, you were expected to go back for seconds and even thirds," relates Rachel. "On each of the major holidays, I could plan on gaining as much as ten pounds." When Rachel was on a "serious" diet, she would begin obsessing about upcoming holidays weeks in advance. "I simply knew that all my good work would be undone—and it always was."

"My mother knew every bite I ate—and every bite I didn't," claims Marc. "She was mortally offended if I skipped some specialty. 'You aren't going to have any?' she would wail. She acted as if she'd been stabbed through the heart!"

"My mother was the worst cook in Kalamazoo, Michigan," recalls Gerry. "But we were still expected to 'feast.'" He has grim memories of overeating on terrible foods. No surprise that Gerry matured into a gourmet chef who loves cooking for his fellow New Yorkers. "And I try not to force-feed anyone," he laughs.

But for many of us, what my brother calls "family state occasions" are no laughing matter. If food equaled love, we could feel neglected and rejected trying to diet amid merry diners—but we found that if we took pen to paper and strategized, we could come up with an approach that worked for us.

In advance of the next holiday, you might want to try writing out the traditional family menu and selecting from its offerings those that are nonthreatening to you. If you can enter the dining room focused on foods that are not triggers for you, you are one step ahead of the game. Most families feature some healthful foods tucked amid the temptations. You might double up on the green beans, take a half cup of wild rice or yams, skip the Jell-O salad with marshmallows, and enjoy some of the meats. It is possible to assemble a nondamaging plate if you pick and choose with care.

TASK

Putting the "Celebration" Back in Holidays

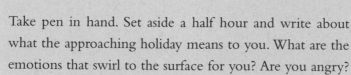

Take pen in hand. Set aside a half hour and write about what the approaching holiday means to you. What are the emotions that swirl to the surface for you? Are you angry? Apprehensive? Excited? How do you relate to those you will be seeing? Are there emotional subtexts that you must grapple with?

Terry, for example, always had to field loaded questions about why she wasn't married yet. The answer: she was gay, but her family strove to deny it. She chronically overate at holidays to defend herself against her family's lobbying that she be something other than who and what she was. Pen in hand, Terry was able to explore—and explode—her family dynamic. She distilled her family's message down to this damning sentence: "Whatever I am is not good enough." I suggested that she reverse the poisonous message by writing a short affirmation to repeat to herself before, during, and after the holiday: "What I am is good enough."

Do you have a negative family message that gets swallowed along with too much food? Can you convert it to a positive, affirmative statement? Is there an action you can take to defuse the family dynamic? You may want to strategize about this with your Body Buddy.

The Food Hangover

Last night I experienced a relapse. I was out to dinner with Domenica, my daughter, and Emma Lively, my musical collaborator. We were eating clean and feeling good about it, until Domenica said she might want to try a bite of dessert. It sounded so innocent. She didn't say, "Let's binge." It was more along the lines of "Let's just have a snibble." But a snibble of what? Domenica chose something called Scarlett O'Hara's Coffee Cantata. It involved coffee ice cream, fresh raspberries, and hot fudge. The waiter brought the delicacy along with a spoon for each of us. Dimly thinking, "This is stupid," I dug in. One bite led to another and then another after that. The ice cream was delicious. Ditto the raspberries and the fudge. I found myself eating more than my fair share. The sugar hit my system like a shock. What was I doing?

What I was doing was relapsing. Before the sundae was halfway devoured, I felt my IQ dipping a few points. I wasn't precisely stoned, more stunned—as though someone had hit me on the head with a small mallet. I was supposed to teach—but teach what? The evening's lesson plan swam in my head. Try as I did, I couldn't focus to think clearly. I felt as though I had had a couple of very stiff drinks.

"Mom, are you OK?" asked my daughter.

"You're not," Emma pronounced.

"I am fine," I protested, but I was not fine, far from it, and I quickly sent up a prayer for help for my foolish self. Call it inspiration or desperation, I dug a notebook out of my briefcase and began scribbling notes to myself about exactly the territory I hoped that the night's class would cover. My handwriting looked loopy. My scrawl seemed drunk. God was going to have to teach the class for me.

"Stick me in the prayer pot," I beseeched Emma and Domenica. "I really can't afford to eat that stuff."

Riding in the cab over to the teaching venue, I felt both drowsy and a little dizzy. I stepped to the curb with care. Inside the building, I went to my classroom and carefully transferred my teaching plan to a large flip chart at the front of the classroom. Once more I noticed that my writing seemed loopy. Did I?

Class was two hours long and I taught it on automatic pilot. I had a feeling of banked alarm—probably the same sort a stoned Vietnam veteran experienced after smoking a joint before his patrol. "God keeps a special eye on fools and drunks," I have often heard said, and I seemed to qualify as both. When class ended, I couldn't wait to dive into a cab and make my way home.

Sleep didn't come to me gently. Instead, it pounced. I slept ten hours, bedeviled by violent dreams. When I woke, my mouth was parched and my head was pounding. Without the aid of any alcohol whatsoever, I had a full-fledged hangover.

TASK

The "Lapse" in Relapse

Take pen to page and re-create for yourself the exact feelings—and circumstances—of your last relapse. Did you, too, get a hangover? Was the food you ate worth the cost it exacted? Did a blocked emotion trigger you to eat, or did your binge seem to come out of nowhere, as mine had?

Very often, writing about a relapse, we see that the "out of nowhere" was really "out of somewhere." Reviewing my own relapse, I see that I was in direct violation of HALT. I was both too hungry and too tired—the week had included a whirlwind teaching trip out to Wyoming and I was still jet-lagged. Further, I was angry that some of my favorite students were cutting the evening's class. Any of these factors were variables enough to make me vulnerable to a slip. And slip I had.

When we slip, we have to pick ourselves up and start again. We need to extend compassion to ourselves. "There, there," we need to say. "Try again." The first thing to do if you have a slip is to forgive yourself—and to know that slips happen to everybody.

I know a five-foot-seven, size-four professional athlete whose last slip consisted of an entire pizza and an entire Sara Lee cake. Does she slip often? No. Does she work many hours a week in the gym? Yes. Did she "get away" with this binge? Yes and no. Alert to the danger she was in, she instantly returned to her Clean Eating track and stepped up her exercise routine. Like me, however, she did experience a physical and psychological hangover. To look at her, she looks perfect—but none of us is perfect.

Identifying Your
Eating Pattern

I never binge," Caroline swore to me. "I never overeat, and I do not deserve to be overweight, so why am I?" I suggested to Caroline that she try keeping a food journal. When she did, she quickly answered her own questions. No, she did not binge. No, she did not overeat. But she did eat nearly constantly. She worked at home, and periodically throughout the day she would go to "check" on her refrigerator, often choosing a small snack— nothing too highly caloric in itself, but her small snacks added up. One hundred fifty calories here, one hundred fifty calories there— in no time she had eaten the caloric equivalent of a nice piece of cheesecake. Caroline's eating pattern is one that I call the "grazer." Like Bessie the cow, she eats more or less constantly. Is it any wonder she carries some extra weight?

Gloria, a fine athlete, eats her food in binges. She often starves herself until late afternoon, when she suddenly consumes a great many high-calorie foods. "I didn't eat any breakfast, and I didn't eat any lunch," she rationalizes. "I deserve to have whatever I want now." Gloria's eating habits are actually bad habits. Her body is constantly ping-ponging between no calories and too many. Psychologically her energy dips match her food consumption. She runs on empty with feelings of stress and loneliness. Then she overeats, bringing on feelings of despair and self-loathing. "I know I should try to eat more regularly, but it's a knack I just haven't mastered yet. Sometimes I seem to myself to be doing just fine on a diet of caffeine and sugar. I love to bake, and I love to taste while I bake. I know this isn't really healthy, but I don't seem motivated to eat earlier in the day. I would say I'm something of a binger, prone to extremes and unable to embrace a healthy moderation." What makes Gloria's case harder and more confusing for herself is the fact that she is actually at an acceptable weight. She yearns to lose another five pounds, but she looks very good exactly as she is, and this fact undercuts her attempts to diet while still setting up in herself a need to diet.

Caitlin is what I call a "snacker." She eats well and carefully, and then rewards herself with a high-calorie snack that undoes all of her good work. "It's as if my virtue lasts only so long," complains Caitlin. "I'm good at breakfast, good at lunch, but by happy hour I'm telling myself I deserve a snack 'just to stabilize my blood sugar.' The problem is, the snacks I choose are high in calories and low in energy. I go for refined sugars and flours, the Krispy Kreme doughnuts of the world. I know I should have a piece of fruit or a container of yogurt, but instead I reward myself with something forbidden." Caitlin's weight hovers about fifteen pounds above her desired weight. While she doesn't think of herself as self-destructive, she is exactly that. "Take yesterday," says Caitlin. "I decided to be more virtuous than usual, and to eat some protein at happy hour. I knew that a small handful of nuts was the right idea, so I made myself a peanut butter and jelly sandwich. I had the nuts, all right, but I also had bread and sugar, spoiling my appetite for dinner, and setting in motion a need for a late-night snack. I can see that I need to eat more regularly if I am ever to learn to eat well."

"I don't have a sugar habit, I have a sugar lifestyle," says Jean, whose "lifestyle" features Coke for breakfast and sugar-coated Cheerios for lunch. "I buy candy by the bag, but I eat it one small piece at a time. I'm never grotesquely overweight, but I'm never thin either. What I am is pale and pasty. I lack the glow of health, and it's no wonder. Nothing healthy touches my lips." Jean is an abusive eater. While her daily caloric intake may not be too high, her sugar habit veers off the charts. High-strung and high-maintenance, Jean has lots of nervous energy but seldom exercises. As a result of her bad habits, Jean looks about a decade older than her calendar age. She feels a decade older, too, beset by myriad aches and pains, troubled by restless sleep and a finicky appetite. Her tastes run to sugar and comfort foods. She does not make the connection that her high sugar intake strips her nerves raw. Instead, she pops another kernel of candy corn and tells herself that she needs the energy to keep going. Jean is what I call a "nibbler." Her type subsists on tiny bites of high-calorie food.

TASK

What Type of Eater Are You?

You may have recognized your eating pattern in the thumb-nail sketches above, or you may have an eating pattern unique to you that has not been covered. Marilyn crams her body with high-protein foods, seldom eating any roughage. A recovering bulimic, she tells herself she is ahead of the game because she no longer binges and purges. Yet, she would be healthier if she were eating a regular regimen of fresh greens. Kathy substitutes caffeine for food. She lives on Starbucks, and whenever her body signals her it is hungry, she doses it with caffeine. "I live on coffee," she laughs nervously. She does everything nervously. Her caffeine intake guarantees that her nervous system overworks itself.

Take pen in hand and describe your eating pattern. Are you a grazer, a binger, a snacker, or a nibbler? How far do you stray from the Clean Eating ideal of three meals and two snacks a day? What is your liquid intake? Sixty-four ounces of water a day is recommended. How close do you come to this goal?

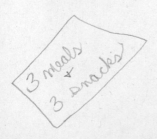

Tabloid Thin

I live in the wrong age," you may catch yourself muttering, eyeing the stick-figured models in a trendy tabloid. "How thin is too thin?" the headlines blare, and you may find yourself answering, "Nothing is thin enough." We are trained by the media to an anorexic ideal of beauty.

"I just have a lucky metabolism," explains Isadora. At five eleven, she sports a size-four figure. "I'm not *really* bulimic," she claims, but she uses the "occasional" purge to regulate her eating.

We need only look at art through the ages to recognize that beauty was once a plump, well-rounded shape. "In another era, I'd have been a red-hot beauty," moans Amanda. She feels her hourglass figure is out of style. No matter that Beyoncé and Jennifer Lopez are admired for their generous curves, Amanda focuses instead on Keira Knightley and Nicole Richie. "I used to run marathons, but even running sixty miles a week didn't change my basic curvaceous structure."

How thin is too thin, and what is thin enough? The media flashes us image after image of wafer-thin waifs, stringier than their string bikinis. Tabloid pages are filled with quick weight-loss programs—pills, potions, and powders that promise a "new you." Collectively we watch with bated breath as Oprah battles pounds. She looks hefty at two hundred, radiant forty pounds thinner, and yet she yearns to be thinner still. 160

Kirstie Alley undertakes a Jenny Craig regimen that sends her weight plummeting and her self-esteem soaring. She promises us she will soon appear on *Oprah* in a bikini. "I'd like to see that," we catch ourselves thinking, and we do. In our national obsession, "fit" and "thin" have come to be synonymous. In our fashion magazines, page after page is devoted to the mincing steps of emaciated young lovelies.

"My arm is the size of her leg," mourns one buxom woman of my acquaintance, pointing to a supermodel spread in *Vogue*. Editors defend the stick-thin images, saying that it is their job to convey fantasy, not reality. But doesn't that fantasy imply an ideal? And hasn't our ideal become far too thin for our own good?

"I hate department-store mirrors," says Abby. "They specialize in cellulite. I can't buy a swim suit. I can't buy an evening gown. What I buy is shapeless, formless, and monochromatic. I know the tricks of dressing in one color, wearing tunics to lengthen my waistline and A-line skirts or wide-legged trousers to diminish my curves. Sometimes I wonder what it would have been like to live in an era when women were frankly buxom. I believe in 'vive la différence,' but I am afraid to dress that way."

"I'm a porker," says Natalie, a fine woman athlete. At five four and one hundred twenty-five pounds, she runs triathlons and is rigorously fit. Still, she takes little joy from her fitness. "I was actually hoping that all that exercise would make me skinny," she admits.

Ours is a distorted lens. We view health and see it as unhealthy. We view dangerously thin and see it as fit. Our standards are set by the media, and we cannot hold them accountable enough for the images that they push. Perhaps we are too brainwashed to even think of holding them accountable.

Bodies come in all shapes and sizes. Not all bodies are intended to be thin. A rounded five-foot-two figure is just as lovely as a five-ten beanstalk—except in the eyes of its owner.

"I am what I am and I have what I have," Carrie, an actress, says of her petite hourglass figure. "I lived in L.A. for five years, and believe me, I learned how to take no for an answer. At five two and one hundred ten pounds, I wasn't what they were looking for. At five ten and one hundred ten pounds, I would have been right up their alley."

"Our ideals of beauty are artificial," says Rosemary, a casting agent. "I cannot tell you how many very talented actresses are considered just a little bit too pudgy when they are really nearly underweight. Time and again I have watched 'thin' win. I don't like it, but it's the reality of the marketplace."

Not all of us live in Hollywood, competing with the Hollywood talent pool to land a job. But the media, and especially the tabloid media, take their cue from Tinseltown. We may live in Omaha, but our idea of beauty still comes to us from Malibu. We read articles detailing how postpregnancy Britney Spears lost twenty-six pounds in just one month. It isn't safe, it isn't healthy, but we yearn to do the same.

The tabloids tell us stories, and we listen to what they say. Katie Holmes shed twenty-three pounds in a month. Kate Hudson shed nearly sixty pounds in three months. Citing a combination of cardio, weight lifting, Pilates, and yoga, these women put in hours daily to recoup the camera-ready, slim, and slight figure they had pre-baby. While pregnancy and consequent weight gain are seen as career catastrophes, nonpregnant women must monitor their figures as well. Weighing in on the skinny side, we have waifs Nicole Richie and Keira Knightley. "I am not anorexic," these women protest, but if they are not anorexic, they are clearly too thin to be healthy. Eyeing a copy of *People* magazine with Mary-Kate Olsen on the cover, a nurse recently remarked, "I don't need to read *People* to decide if she's anorexic." Anorexic or not, Olsen is envied and emulated, proving again the adage that a woman can never be too thin or too rich.

It is hard work detoxing from media saturation. It takes independent thinking to decide for ourselves that plump may be more pleasing than skinny. We have a few examples of curvaceous figures grabbing the spotlight. Jennifer Lopez with her famous "booty" made the derriere an erogenous zone. Beyoncé, with curves in places where many women have no places, proved that pulchritude and amplitude could go hand in hand.

Aurora, a red-haired siren with a chassis Jessica Rabbit might envy, tells the story of her time in Hollywood. "How to put this modestly? I was used to thinking of myself as a good-looking woman, and men had always seemed to do the same. In both London and New York, I worked frequently, both in theater and in film. At my agent's suggestion, I decided to try Hollywood. First they wanted me to dye my signature red hair platinum; next, they wanted me to 'come down' a couple of dress sizes. I was so desperate to make it that I did dye my hair, and I did diet. California is the land of great produce, and I lived on salads. I quickly found that I was a blond bitch, deprived of my necessary nutrients. When I finally got work, blond bitch is how they cast me, and I spent three full years trying to live out that image. It was only when I fell in love with a Latin who liked a little flesh on his women that I snapped to and realized I had sold myself out. Now I'm red-haired, fifteen pounds heavier, and working in the industry, but as a screenwriter, not an actor. I simply couldn't take the pressure to conform."

TASK

What Is Your Ideal Beauty?

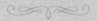

Do you have a well-rounded view of beauty, or do you find yourself falling prey to media manipulation? Collect ten fashion magazines. Buy a piece of poster board and some glue. For one half hour, sort through your magazine stash, pulling any image that speaks to you of feminine beauty. At the end of a half hour, paste your images in place. What do you see? Do you have an attainable sense of beauty, or are you placing yourself out of the ballpark by coveting the stick-thin figure that will never be yours? Beauty is made of so many factors—a good head of hair, a rounded eye, a smiling lip, a graceful neck, a bust and hips that are ample. Are you able to swim against the media tide? Are you able to craft for yourself a sense of style and beauty that may not match the anorexic norm we are asked to buy into?

Scaling the Scale

Mary-Louise seems like a healthy and normal woman. Her body is a healthy and normal weight; her clothes are stylish and well fitted. Her persona is appealing, so what's wrong with this picture? Mary-Louise wakes every morning with a dread of the scale she keeps tucked just under her bed. A quick trip to the bathroom and then she steps onto her wafer-thin, digital scale. There, in pounds and ounces, she receives her self-image for the day. Has she gained or lost weight overnight? Did the Chinese food she so enjoyed cause her to bloat? What does the scale have to say?

"I know I shouldn't weigh myself every day. I know it's probably obsessive. I know my weight may vary by as much as five pounds, depending on what I ate the night before, but I just can't help myself. I want to know the truth, and yet I know that the number given to me by the scale often is not the truth, that I may be carrying water weight or a few premenstrual pounds."

If her scale is up, Mary-Louise finds that her mood plummets straight down. If her scale is down, her mood skitters skyward.

Never pausing to ask, "How do I really look today?" she instead takes the scale's word for it. She is "thin enough" or not.

"Too often, I'm an 'or not,' " says Mary-Louise. "There are five elusive pounds that I keep chasing, telling myself that if I just reach that goal weight, my life will be perfect, my insecurities will disappear, and my clothes will look better than ever. I don't know why I focus so on clothes. What I'm really asking the scale is 'how would I look stark naked?' I keep waiting to be thin enough to have a lover."

Craving intimacy, we pursue an impossible goal through harsh regimens and exercise rather than by working on self-acceptance, on the idea that we may be fine just as we are. We pursue instead an illusory ideal. We will be fine "when . . ." When we are a size eight? A size six? A size four? I know women who wear a size two and still complain they are chubby. They reinforce this perception by stepping daily onto their scales.

"My scale is my conscience," claims Glenda. "I eat a peanut-brittle candy bar and wait for my scale to tell me the damage. Sometimes, if I'm walking on the treadmill regularly enough, I seem to get away with a mini binge. But the minute the scale says no, no, I'm back to starvation rations."

"Think of the scale as a tough-love friend," one nutritionist warns. "It will give you the news, but it's usually the bad news." Why not try weighing once weekly? Even more radical, why not try weighing once a month? The scale then becomes an emergency net, not a daily companion.

"My clothes are actually the most accurate way for me to gauge my size," says Jeanette. "If my clothes have a loose, easy fit, I know

I'm on the right track. If my clothes feel too tight or too small, I'm in trouble."

As we increase our exercise and speed up our metabolism, we tend to lose bulk. Muscle is more compact than fat. We may change an entire dress size, or even two, without budging the needle on the scale.

"I knew my diet was succeeding when I began to be able to fit into my old clothes," says Judith. "I thanked my lucky stars that I had not discarded them."

Scaling back on our use of the scale can be a positive choice. Freed from the tyranny of numbers, we begin instead to focus on ourselves and our own perceptions. We know that if we eat clean, weight loss will follow. When we release ourselves from the daily use of the scale, we find ourselves able to embrace a more "easy does it" approach to weight loss. We begin to see that as long as we are moving in the right direction, the speed at which we reach our destination matters less.

"I try to wear my food plan like a loose garment," declares Antonia. She no longer weighs herself daily; instead, she uses the fit of her clothes to tell her her progress.

The healthiest way to view our relationship to food is to see it in terms of progress, not perfection. Many of us have for many years endured a toxic relationship to our food. Now we are eating more healthfully, if not perfectly. This is progress, and it is progress with which we must learn to be satisfied.

"I wanted to take my scale outside and shoot it," exclaims Dee Dee. "It was really a device of torture for me. No matter how thin I became, I always wanted to be just a little thinner. No matter what number flashed on the scale, I wished for a lower one. Obsessed with weight loss instead of with physical fitness, I failed to congratulate myself on my wins, and once I began eating clean, there were many wins. I became leaner and more fit; my thinking around food became far more clear and less obsessive; what I ate became fuel for what I was trying to do—not my entire identity. Now I weigh myself once a month—if I remember. I use the scale simply to corroborate my perceptions. It's now my servant, not my master."

TASK

Scale Back on Your Scale

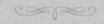

If your scale enjoys center stage in your bathroom or your bedroom, if you are unable to let a day pass by without setting foot on it, the time has come to retire your scale from its place of prominence. If you panic at the thought of not checking in, know that this panic will pass. It is far healthier to focus on right eating and right exercise than it is to focus on a certain number. You may wish to place your scale in a closet or under your bed—"out of sight, out of mind." For some of us this is a terrifying idea. We are addicted to weighing ourselves. We are habituated to the adrenaline rush of facing the bad news. We do not trust ourselves or our own perceptions.

"How can I trust myself?" asks Charlene. "I lie to myself constantly about food. I tell myself I'll eat just a bite, then I'm off to the races on a binge. I feel the scale is all that stands between me and disaster. I can only imagine what would happen if I tried to go a month without its input."

If you are eating clean, you will lose weight. It will come off slowly and gradually, but it will come off. By resigning from the daily weigh-in, you resign from self-punishment. It puts your weight squarely back between you and a higher power.

Tell yourself you will weigh yourself again one month from today. Trust yourself and your newly formed eating habits to move your body in the direction of optimum health.

Relapse

For many of us, a diet is an exercise in futility and self-flagellation. We set a plan in motion and then we sabotage it. We take a step toward our goal and then we relapse. We undo the good we've done.

I was doing fine yesterday until nine at night. That's when I decided to go to a diner to have a cup of hot tea and a nice piece of cherry pie. What's wrong with a little cherry pie? my thinking ran. After all, it's fruit! How fattening can it really be? And so, telling myself it wasn't *really* fattening—meaning not as fattening as molten chocolate cake, for example, or a banana split— I ate the cherry pie. You know how it is with cherry pie. It's hard to get a really good piece. And this piece was worse than mediocre. The filling was gelid, the cherries were few and far between, the crust was stale. For dessert at a good diner, it was certainly no advertisement for their fare. I came home feeling buzzed from the sugar, and I slept poorly as a result. When I woke up this morning, I had a full-fledged sugar hangover. Yes, I had had a relapse.

"Just a little relapse," I wanted to say. But that is what all relapses advertise themselves as. It doesn't take much to undo a good day's eating. A slice of pie, a wedge of cheesecake, a few homemade cookies. Surely, we reason, after a day of virtue we deserve a treat.

A treat is just a relapse in sheep's clothing. We treat ourselves to mashed potatoes instead of zucchini. We treat ourselves to two dinner rolls with butter. We treat ourselves—we treat ourselves badly! We go for the quick fix of a trigger food, pulling the trigger on our own eating sobriety.

"I've been in Overeaters Anonymous off and on for twenty years. I've spent years on the Gray Sheet. I've answered the questionnaires from HOW. I've been abstinent and I've been thin, sometimes too thin. My sponsor told me not to be so rigid, but for me it's all or nothing. If I slip on a piece of cake, I want the corner piece with all the frosting." So states Suzanne, emphatically. To anyone's eye but her own, Suzanne is thin, almost too thin. She keeps a treadmill in her bedroom and runs on it nightly, doubling her efforts when she has relapsed.

"I want to lose another twenty pounds," Suzanne announces. She plucks at her waistline, where there is barely an inch of pinch. "Maybe I'm a little bit obsessive, maybe I take things too far. Maybe I should try for moderation. . . ." Her voice trails off.

There is no maybe about it. Moderation would release Suzanne from the bondage of obsession about her weight. If she could learn not to eat the corner piece, she would be far ahead of the game. A wise diet, like South Beach, allows for the fact that we will occasionally slip from our grid and overeat. A steady exercise regimen is the best defense against such mini relapses. A recent *New York Times* article pinpointed the positive value of exercise after a heavy meal. A good walk, a visit to the treadmill or the

StairMaster, a half hour on the stationary bike—all of these are fine ammunition in our war with overweight. And it is a war.

"I do it strictly by calories," claims Janice. "If I relapse by three hundred fifty calories, I must up my exercise by three hundred fifty calories. This means I can have pancakes for breakfast if I hit the treadmill soon after."

What doesn't work for most of us is the relapse that goes unrepented. The piece of pie that isn't addressed by exercise becomes the extra inch we wear on our derriere.

"I don't believe I'm helpless about relapses," argues Mary defiantly. "When I get the urge to eat, I drink water instead. I have found that two eight-ounce glasses of water will usually kill my appetite for self-destruction. I keep water in my refrigerator so that when I am tempted I can reach for water instead."

To many of us, water sounds unappealing—tasteless, flat, even repellent. There are now on the market many fruit-flavored waters that can trick our taste buds into submission.

"I drink lemon and raspberry splash," says Carla. "I use it to trick myself. Let's say I want to eat all the candy corn left over from Halloween. I tell myself, four bottles of water, and then I have permission to binge. By the third bottle, I've always lost my taste for misadventure."

Some of us keep water stations scattered throughout the house—a six-pack of water next to the bedside reading station, a six-pack by the TV, another six-pack in the dining room, a refrigerator full.

"I look at water as my insurance policy against a bad relapse," says Anna. "I don't know what it is about two glasses of water that takes all the fun out of a candy bar or a scoop of ice cream, but it does. I once tried three glasses of water and a helping of Dulce de Leche. I couldn't even clean the bowl. That's what I call a miracle."

In dealing with our tendency to relapse, most of us need little miracles. The trick for many of us is how to stop before we have a full-fledged binge. This is where our journal and the four questions come in handy. "Am I hungry?" we ask, and the answer is often, "No, but I am restless." Next we ask, "Is this what I want to eat? Is this what I want to eat now? Is there something else I can eat instead?" Lo and behold, our high-caloric binge mysteriously fades into a cup of diet Jell-O or a Fuji apple and a slice of sharp cheddar cheese.

"Is there something else that I can do instead of eat?" We eventually learn to ask ourselves a fifth question. A half hour's needlepoint becomes the substitution for a big bowl of buttered popcorn or bag of potato chips. Television doesn't need to be a cue for overeating. We often find we just need something in our lap. Needlepoint, a crossword puzzle, even a cozy pillow.

"My dog gets a lot more affection now that I've given up my popcorn habit," says Karen.

TASK

Take a Look at Your Relapses

Cue up a piece of relaxing music. Curl up on the couch and take pen in hand. How do you relapse, and why? Get the details on paper. Do you relapse like I do, in many small ways? Or do you relapse in large ways? Do you relapse seldom or often? What foods are your favorite relapse foods? Must you keep them in your house? Have you tried the water trick? Does it work for you? Is there a hobby that appeals to you that you could use to fill your evening eating hours? Are you able to cancel out your relapse with effective exercise? Does writing down your food and using the four questions help you to halt a relapse midstream, or avoid one altogether?

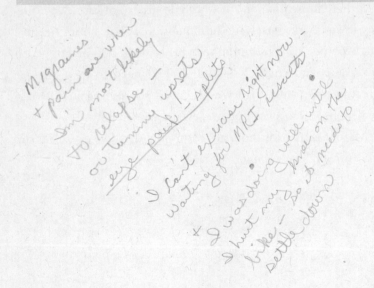

Snack Smart

I have one basic problem with dieting," says Janet, "I love food."
Most of us love food. Most of us love food too much. Faced
with going without, we are afraid of our feelings. "I'll feel so miserable! I'll feel so deprived! I'll feel so . . ." I'll feel, period. Food
is a powerful sedative. We administer food as we would a medicine. Asked to go too long between meals, we find our moods soar
and plummet with our blood sugar. In order for a diet to work for
us, we need to be able to eat—eat something! The something that
we need to eat is a snack. While some successful diets have been
built on three square meals and nothing in between, more successful diets are built on the acknowledgment that we need snacks
between meals. But those snacks cannot be mini meals—they need
to be snacks, lower in caloric content and in volume than a real
meal. Recovering alcoholics are often told to snack on a high-
protein food like trail mix during happy hour. As one wag put it,
"There's nothing wrong with my blood sugar that a couple drinks
wouldn't fix—except they'd kill me." So almonds, cashews,
peanuts, and raisins replace Margaritaville. Snack in hand, the sober
alcoholic makes it safely to the evening meal.

For those of us who are not alcoholic, going too long without food may be merely difficult, not dangerous. But difficult is the undoing of a diet, and so we do well to plan carefully to allow for snacks. "I need protein!" exclaims Megan, a fit young athlete who burns calories at a high rate. "In between meals, I snack on yogurt, nuts, or sandwich meats. My favorite snack is homemade tuna salad. I find that a scoop of tuna curbs my appetite just the right amount, and keeps my energy up."

Michael also chooses a high-protein snack. In his prejournaling days, he was a cereal junkie. Midway through the afternoon, he would eat a big bowl of sugary cereal. "I ate like a kindergarten kid," Michael recalls. "I'd get a quick rush of well-being from my snack, but it wasn't enough to really tide me over until dinner. I often found myself eating a second snack—make that two handfuls of dry cereal. This second snack ruined my appetite for dinner and left me feeling sluggish."

Once he undertook journaling and the four questions, Michael began to make smart snacking substitutions. In place of sugary cereal, he ate yogurt with fresh fruit. Instead of needing a second snack, he found himself able to cruise successfully on one.

"I realized that in late afternoon I often wasn't really hungry, I was bored or restless, or stressed by the events of my day. I found that by making myself a nice cup of hot tea, I could unwind a little. At the very least, I kept my mood and my weight from escalating."

"My refrigerator is a snacker's paradise," claims Carlotta. "I have almonds, string cheese, fresh chopped vegetables, fresh fruit, yogurts, lox, and diet Jell-O and puddings. Nowadays it's a question of which treat I should enjoy. All of my snacks are low calorie and high energy. I find I make it through the late-afternoon blahs without turning blue."

The secret to successful snacking is shrewd shopping. As Carlotta explains: "All of my snacks appeal to me." She shops as carefully for her snacks as she does for her entrees, knowing that it is a habit of wrong snacking that has sabotaged her in the past.

TASK

Clean and Stock Your Refrigerator

Begin by taking everything out—that's everything—and giving your refrigerator a thorough, hygienic scrubbing. A clean refrigerator is an appetizing refrigerator. Remember that your diet is not about not eating, it is about eating well.

Now take yourself shopping. Allow yourself to buy "treats"—fresh strawberries, raspberries, blueberries, good Greek yogurt, low-fat string cheese, peaches, plums, and some good, solid protein like tuna fish, lox, or sliced turkey. Don't forget your sweet tooth—buy diet Jell-O and low-calorie puddings. Checking the calorie count, you may want to add hummus or baba ghanoush. Low-fat cottage cheese is another snack favorite, with a sprinkling of cinnamon. Treat yourself the way you would treat a new lover. Buy yourself low-fat but delicious delicacies. *Bon appétit!*

Night Eating

Once more, it's like something out of a science-fiction movie—every night at about ten o'clock, my refrigerator begins to glow. It exudes a heavenly light. It speaks in an angelic whisper. It says, "Just a bite! You've been so good all day. Surely you deserve a bedtime snack?" And so I pad to the kitchen, swing open the refrigerator door, and survey the contents. The four questions swing briefly to mind, but I'm not listening to them. The answer to question number one, "Am I hungry?" is, of course, "No, not really." But I don't want this information. What I want is a bedtime snack.

Mick often works double shifts at the steak house. All day long he is surrounded by delicious, high-quality food, and all day long he dodges temptation. Everyone at the job knows that Mick is on a diet. What they don't know is that he routinely sabotages that diet every night on his way home from work.

"I tell myself that I've been good all day," says Mick. "I tell myself that riding my bike to work burns calories. I tell myself that since I'm so good, I deserve a treat, and then I pull my bike into

Wendy's and order a double cheeseburger with fries. Needless to say, my diet goes right out the window. I consume a full day's calories every night at midnight. I tell myself I deserve the treat, but the truth is I'm treating myself badly."

Many of us, like Mick, tell ourselves that our nighttime eating is just a harmless treat. We would be horrified if anyone accused us of being self-destructive, and yet we *are* self-destructive.

"I don't really live in my body, I just visit it," laughs Amy, a pretty woman forty pounds overweight. She tries to tell herself it's "not spiritual" to focus on the body. Instead, she tries to "transcend" her extra weight. She dresses in flowing robes and exudes an "earth mother" calm—but calm is far from how she feels when she compares herself to other, right-size women.

"I can't believe how jealous I am," moans Amy. "I really resent my girlfriends and their girlish figures. I would go so far as to say I almost *hate* my closest friend, who seems to be able to eat anything and never gain an ounce. She's very sweet about my own weight. She always tells me I'm beautiful, that I have a pretty face. That makes me even madder. I feel like she's helping me to rationalize, and that's not true friendship."

But what *is* true friendship? Do we really want our friends to say, "Yes, you're gaining weight, and it doesn't look good." Do we want our friends to count calories for us? Most of us secretly prefer enablers, those friends who help us to gain weight by offering to share their sweet potato pie, or "just a few bites" of their raspberry crème brûlée.

"You're very pretty," Amy's enabler always tells her. She doesn't add the word "still," although she certainly could. At one hundred thirty-five pounds Amy was a dazzling woman. At one hundred seventy-five pounds she is pleasantly plump, and there's nothing too pleasant about it.

"I'm good during the day," Amy claims, "but every night I reach for comfort food. I don't want to be alone, I don't want to be lonely, and so I cue up a romantic comedy and butter up a big batch of popcorn."

If she were able to be honest with herself, Amy would face her yearning for an intimate relationship. But honesty is subverted by her nightly eating. While candor would tell us that something is wrong and we are eating to medicate that something, rationalization tells us nothing is really wrong, and that we deserve a treat after a long day of virtue.

"I swear to God, I have to eat in order to be able to sleep," asserts Josh, a hard-driven executive who carries an extra twenty-five pounds around his ever-expanding waist. His days are so stress ridden, the demands on his time and attention are so intense, his late-night malted milks pose as mere comfort food, and he rationalizes them to himself that they are "healthy"—he needs the calcium, after all.

Many of us destroy a day's good eating with our late-night binges. We tell ourselves that such lapses are actually medicinal. "It's better than a sleeping pill," we say of our bowl of vanilla Häagen-Dazs. "It reminds me of Mom," we say of our snack of cookies and milk. What we are looking for is a combination of safety and comfort. These qualities can come to us through channels other than eating.

Marion, a high-powered ad executive, learned that she could wind down at night by listening to soothing music for half an hour. "I call it my safety music," Marion says, and she cues up a selection, instead of scooping the Ben and Jerry's that waits in her freezer.

"I use both music and incense," says Suzanne. "It may sound bizarre, but I'm trying to avoid a late-night bowl of cereal. My very favorite is oatmeal with brown sugar, butter, and cream. Instead, I make myself a cup of chamomile tea and lay back to listen to celestial music and inhale the heavenly fragrance of Nag Champa incense."

"Too much virtue is too much virtue," protests Krissy, who is unwilling to give up her late-night snack. "I crave something sweet at night, and so I make myself a cup of cocoa using Valrhona cocoa powder, skim milk, and Splenda. I find it better to 'fool' my sweet tooth than to try to avoid it altogether. I try to make a smart choice, using the skim milk and Splenda to avoid high-caloric intake." For most of us, it all comes back to willingness. Are we willing to strategize around our late-night eating? First, we must admit that we do have a problem. Second, we must admit that we are not going to succeed at magically giving up our nocturnal treat. We do best to plan a snack that does the least amount of damage. We may resent it, but we *can* work with the four questions. Diet Jell-O in the place of Häagen-Dazs may seem like a sorry compromise, but it's actually "good enough."

Speaking for myself, I had to learn that "good enough" *was* good enough. In place of cherry-almond cake, I could make do with two containers of diet cherry Jell-O, or a bowl of sliced strawberries with fat-free half-and-half. Like Krissy, I could make a cup of diet hot cocoa. I could even cue up some safety music and sip a soothing cup of tea.

"To hell with soothing," says Kitty, who keeps a treadmill in her bedroom. "Exercise kills appetite. When I get a late-night craving, I climb on my treadmill. I find that after running a mile, my appetite diminishes. I believe in fighting fire with fire."

TASK

Find Something New to Do

Let me be blunt: if we have eaten well during the day, we are rarely *really* hungry at night. Instead, we are using food as a sedative to medicate our unruly emotions. Take pen in hand. Number from one to ten. List ten activities you *could* undertake instead of nighttime eating.

For example:

1. Leave a message on my Body Buddy's machine that I am tempted to eat.
2. Make a gratitude list.
3. Make a friendship list, naming all those to whom I feel close.
4. Organize my closet.
5. Scrub my bathroom.
6. Polish my shoes.
7. Clean my makeup brushes and hairbrushes.
8. Take a hot shower and brush and floss my teeth.

9. Make a hot cup of tea.
10. Make a hot cup of diet cocoa (2 heaping table-spoons highest-quality cocoa powder [like Val-rhona], 1 cup skim milk, Splenda to taste).

Post this list on your refrigerator.

Food as Sedative

Most of us like to think that we live to the fullest, finding a sense of adventure in every moment. If we are honest, this is actually an ideal, not a reality, and many of us feel a sense of dissatisfaction when we scrutinize our lives closely. Like that old Peggy Lee song "Is That All There Is?" we sense that there *must* be more to life than we are experiencing. What's wrong? we wonder, feeling a sense of unease. "Something's bugging me," we may say aloud, but we don't know just what. "If only I could get to the bottom of this," we may muse, but instead of digging into our psyches, we open the door to the refrigerator.

"I wouldn't say that food kept me shallow," says Angela, "but it actually did. Whenever I felt the stirrings to create something, I took them as hunger pangs. Rather than write a new song, I would head for the freezer. After a bowl of Rocky Road, I felt no need to create. In fact, I felt no needs, period. Ice cream worked as a sedative."

If we are honest, many of us can admit that we've used food as a sedative. Not all food, of course, not the food we take in during a day's Clean Eating, but the extra food that seems to sneak in around the edges—the late-night snacks, the sugary or salty treats, the "little somethings" we give to ourselves when we experience a moment of boredom, restlessness, or irritability.

"I'll get back to it in a moment," we think as we abandon a creative project or a tricky piece of business and retreat to nibbling on an unneeded snack. But very often the snack derails our train of thought, and we do not get back to what we were working on. Instead, we take a detour, telling ourselves we've been productive enough for the day.

But what does productive enough really mean? Are we living up to our potential? Do we fill each day with small but worthy accomplishments, or do we procrastinate, postpone, avoid, and evade?

"I was good for about an hour and a half," recalls Rebecca. "If I got back from lunch at one-thirty, I could work until about three, and then my clock would start ticking, telling me it was time to eat something else. Our office was often overflowing with snack foods. I wasn't the only one using food as a crutch to get through my workday."

In cases like this, the four questions can bring a Snack Attack to a screeching halt. Am I hungry? you ask yourself, and the honest answer is no. You aren't hungry. Rather, you feel overwhelmed by taking the next right step. It seems so much easier to snack than it does to draft the difficult office memo.

Food is a sedative. We use it to block our feelings of discomfort. We use it to block our feelings, period. Rather than buckle down and accomplish the difficult piece of work that looms just ahead, we scoop up a snack and tell ourselves the work can wait until tomorrow—which it often can.

"I wasn't very efficient," admits Tracy. "I was thirty pounds overweight, and most of that weight came from office snacking. I liked to tell myself I was a good employee, but was I? When I gave up my habit of office Snack Attacks, I became far more productive. My productivity increased even as my weight decreased. 'You're doing something right,' my boss told me, and awarded me a raise. Without overeating, I suddenly had the energy to tackle projects I had long delayed."

If many of us use food as a sedative on the job, many more of us use food as a sedative once we're home from the office. A quick stop at a pizza parlor or a trip to a deli for a high-powered energy drink, and we have fueled ourselves up for our trip home, where we will eat dinner.

"I would eat while I was waiting to eat," says Patricia. "I would put a quick meal in the microwave, but then I would graze through the refrigerator, looking for something to eat while my meal was nuking."

Like Patricia, many of us eat more or less constantly. We have our official meals and our official snacks, and then we have all the food we consume in addition. Writing in our food journals often gives us our first clarity as to just how much, and just how often we really eat. "Do I have to record *everything*?" we whine, noting that we've gone back for a second handful of high-caloric nuts.

"My God, I was like a cow, always grazing!" exclaimed Carolyn. "My apartment was filled with little dishes and trays, all holding treats for the company that never came. I was the company that enjoyed the sugarcoated almonds, the toffee twists, and the party-colored jelly beans. At Halloween I was the trick-or-treater who needed to have plenty of candy for any visitors."

Like Carolyn, many of us are mindless snackers, grazing our way through our days and our nights, scooping up something tasty to divert ourselves from our uncomfortable feelings.

"As long as I overate, I underfelt," says Josh. It helps to think of our emotions as being like a keyboard, running from bass to treble, from low to high. Most of us have just a few notes we are comfortable with, and we eat to block the others.

"I was astounded by how *many* emotions I had," relates Isabella. "I learned that I had many feelings, and that my feelings could come and go with lightning speed. 'This too shall pass,' my 12-step sponsor often told me, and I learned that she was right. Feelings were not facts, they were simply feelings, and feelings pass."

For most of us, the variety of our feelings is a revelation. Once we become accustomed to the change, it is as if our lives have gone from black-and-white to Technicolor. Without food as a sedative, our lives become vivid, active, and highly enjoyable. Where before we told ourselves food was the reward, we now learn that life itself is.

TASK

You Take a Sedative Because . . .

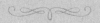

Once we recognize that food is a powerful sedative, we need to ask ourselves what feelings we are trying to sedate.

Take pen in hand and number from one to five. Finish the following phrase:

If I let myself admit it, I feel sad that . . . *I can't exercise & swim :)* [handwritten]

Take pen in hand again. Number from one to five. Finish the following phrase:

If I let myself admit it, I feel mad that . . . *I don't do the right things* [handwritten]

Take pen in hand a third time. Number from one to five. Finish the following phrase:

If I let myself admit it, I feel bad that . . . *I don't do the right things* [handwritten]

What you have just written is known in 12-step parlance as a spot-check inventory. If you suspect that you regularly use food as a sedative, then you should regularly write nightly inventory. If you do so, you will rapidly become more intimate with yourself and more authentic in your exchanges with others.

Food as High

For many of us, food is distinctly mood-altering. We get high from eating certain foods. Sometimes we get high simply from eating. Rather than feel our feelings in all their intensity and variability, we use food to feel different—and, temporarily, better. Although we may know we shouldn't, we seek out those foods that enter our system with a shock. We go for the hot fudge sundae, or the handful of homemade chocolate chip cookies. We're not necessarily trying to block bad feelings; we're trying instead to feel good ones.

Jenny looks forward to a meal of fish and chips, banana pudding, and Coca-Cola—salt, grease, and sugar. "Yum!" she says, anticipating her binge. She looks forward to getting high—high on food. Sure, she will need to diet for a couple of days afterward, but to her the spree is worth it.

The spree is also worth it to Joe, who "knows better" but periodically acts out with the comfort foods from his childhood. "Every day I go for a fancy business lunch—some minute portion of protein on a lettuce leaf. It's all very chic, but it's not very satisfying. What I crave is macaroni and cheese or chicken potpie. I like home fries and malted milks. I hate to admit it, but I'm a diner kind of guy."

Sometimes, when Joe's job becomes too stressful, he plans a binge. Half the fun of bingeing lies in anticipating the binge. Prone to overweight, Joe knows that the foods he loves are "illegal," but that does not stop him. Accustomed to carrying an extra twenty-five pounds, he rationalizes that weight comes with age, not with his ping-pong dieting. Then, too, there is the fact of his traveling for work. Everyone knows how hard it is to maintain a diet on the road. So Joe sets himself up for a spree of his favorite comfort foods—room service fried chicken, room service pasta (as close as he can get to macaroni and cheese), room service desserts.

"It's hard enough being on the road without being on a diet too," says Joe. He always comes home up a few pounds, and he's defensive about his love handles.

"My partner and I no longer tell each other what the scale tells us. After all, we're in it for better or for worse."

Joe tries every new diet that is published. He has an entire library of weight-loss books, but he lacks the willpower to use them.

"Maybe I'm a big baby," Joe says. "Maybe I just want things my way. Maybe if I tried writing about some of this, I might get somewhere. What do you think?"

TASK

What Are Your Comfort Foods?

Take pen in hand. Number from one to five. List your top five comfort foods. Can any of them reasonably be included in your food plan? Can you eat "lean" instead of merely clean, and hoard enough calories to indulge yourself?

Madeline, a svelte New Yorker, discovered that two days of eating salad Niçoise gave her permission for an evening of fish and chips. "I was probably pushing it when I ate the fried Mars bar for dessert," she laughs, but she upped her exercise quotient to offset the offending calories.

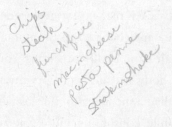

chips
steak
french fries
mac n cheese
pasta penne
steak n shake

A Calorie

Is a Calorie

*F*or optimum weight loss, it's best to eat clean—that is, to shape
your diet so that refined sugars, flours, and starches are kept
to a minimum. Eating clean reduces cravings. Three days off sugar,
and you no longer lust after sweets. A piece of fruit will satisfy what
used to be a candy-bar craving.

A calorie is a calorie, whether it comes from protein, fat, or carbohydrates. Fat, however, contains twice as many calories per gram
as protein or carbohydrates. Your basal metabolic rate is the amount
of calories you need to support your basic bodily functions. Your
BMR is determined by both your body size and its composition.
A large person has a higher BMR than a small person. This is why
a large person can lose weight while consuming more calories
than a small person.

Without exercising, an average-size woman would have to eat
a mere thousand calories a day in order to lose two pounds a
week. By adding exercise to the dietary regimen, that same woman
could eat as much as 1400 calories and still lose weight at the
same rate. In other words, moderate exercise can mark the differ-

ence between a "too difficult" diet and the ideal of bearable Clean Eating.

There's no magic. If you are an average woman, you need to eat approximately 1900 calories a day to maintain your weight. If you eat 1400 calories a day, even if it's all fried Mars bars, you will still lose a pound a week. If you exercise 500 calories per day, you will lose two pounds a week. So why not live on sugar, sugar, sugar? Why not eat candy corn and tote up your calories? The answer, again, is simple: Good eating means good health.

Phyllis is skinny as a racehorse but lives on diet Coke and menthol cigarettes. She has a chronic cough, which she ignores, and she applies her makeup skillfully to offset the pallor of her skin. Phyllis is chicly thin, but she is not fit. Her diet undermines her health rather than supporting it.

"I always thought I ate pretty well," says Peggy, who undertook journaling to lose a stubborn ten pounds she could not shake. "When I began journaling, I was appalled to see what my food choices really were. I lived on caffeine and high-protein, high-fat meals. It's a wonder I didn't have heart or cholesterol problems."

Many of us find, in recording our food, that we use our whole day's caloric allotment long before our day is through. A couple of cocktails at happy hour and a hamburger finds us hungry and grazing at bedtime.

"My extra ten pounds were all nighttime eating," claims Peggy. "I had to take a hard line with myself. I found that by giving up my cocktails, I was able to conserve calories enough for a bedtime snack. All it took was a little discipline—that, and the willingness to stop rationalizing."

For many of us, the journal is a real eye-opener. We think we know how we eat and how we live until we see our patterns in black and white. All too many of us skimp on breakfast, grabbing a quick container of yogurt, telling ourselves it's low in calories and good for us, although we often choose high-sugar brands. For some of us, the afternoon highball is our downfall. Instead of one or two drinks, we routinely consume four, and those drinks are often oversize.

A calorie may be a calorie, but if too many of our calories come from alcohol, we've got a problem. If too many of our calories come from sugar we've got a problem. If too many of our calories come from fat or protein, we've also got a problem. Clean Eating is balanced eating—that means no bingeing at any point on the compass.

Robert is a success story. A chubby child, he grew up plagued by overweight, and determined to fight it. He attended diet camps. He attended Weight Watchers while still in his teens. Nothing seemed to work well enough—every calorie that touched his lips turned to fat. He was unhappy and unconscious, until he stumbled upon the rudiments of Clean Eating. For fifteen years now Robert has maintained his goal weight. He does it not by fad diets, and not by deprivation, but by Clean Eating with a hawk's eye on portion control. Refined sugars, refined flours, fatty and too-high-protein foods are all nos on Robert's regimen. A creative man, he discovered that as his creativity went up, his weight went down. Now, in addition to regular exercise, he sets a regular regimen of playing his guitar and singing. "I knew all about the joy of eating," says Robert. "Food was my first love. What I needed to do was learn how to love myself through Clean Eating, and how to love the many other delights life had to offer. Now, instead of diet camp, I go to fiddle camp. Saturday mornings you will find me tap dancing. Yes, I will eat a piece of chocolate pistachio cake, but it's a very small piece, and I up my exercise afterward." No one loved food more than Robert, and to hear him tell it, this is still the case. He has a highly developed palate, and these days enjoys a part-time job as a taster for a high-end bakery, where he is instrumental in forging the delicacies of the chef.

"I never thought I'd be paid to eat," Robert laughs, "but that is the reward for me of healthful eating. The calories I consume all come from quality sources, and I enjoy very good health now that I feed myself with loving care."

TASK

Making a Portion Pie

Take pen in hand. Draw a circle. Divide the circle into six wedges. Label those wedges protein, fat, carbohydrate, water, fruits and vegetables, and junk food. Now place a dot indicating whether you do well or poorly at consuming in this category. Toward the center is poorly, toward the outer rim is well. Does your food plan resemble a well-balanced mandala, or is it a lopsided, tortured tarantula? Are you imbibing the ideal of sixty-four ounces of water daily? Many of us are lucky if we consume eight. Another frequently abused wedge is the slice for fruits and vegetables. Most people eat few raw foods despite their many health benefits. The wedge for carbohydrates is often maxed out. Believe it or not, it's actually okay to eat a meal without consuming bread and butter. Another high-point offender is the protein wedge. We eat red meat, lots of it, telling ourselves that as long as it's lean it's healthy. This can be too much of a good thing. We're low on chicken, and even lower on fish, although we dimly know that salmon is good for us. The junk food wedge is frequently the slice where many of us lie just a little. We eat junk food daily, unlike fruits and vegetables. But we are often reluctant to acknowledge just how high a percentage of our food intake is empty calories. A late-night snack of pretzels or nuts often escapes our radar altogether.

Look at your portion pie. Work honestly with your own feedback. Trust yourself. Do not wait. Today is the day to start drinking more water. Today is a fine day to snack on fruits and vegetables. Right where you are is the very place to begin.

Exercise

Victoria is a small, curvy brunette. If you ask her, she's too curvy. At five feet one, she always carries an extra five to ten pounds—pounds that a taller person could get away with. For Victoria, the difference between plump and pleasing is very simple: Did she get to the gym? Like many of us, Victoria tends to carry water weight. But a session on the treadmill, the StairMaster, or the stationary bike, and the bloat starts to melt away. Within three days of recommitting to the gym, Victoria can sense a difference. When she is flirted with by the cute trainer, she lightly flirts back. It's no longer a shock that someone finds her attractive. With exercise, Victoria finds herself attractive.

"My baggy clothes are the first things to go," Victoria laughs. "When I'm not exercising, I hide out in them. I wear several sizes too large for me. I tell myself this makes me look slimmer, but it actually makes me look plump."

After a few days in the gym, Victoria starts to sport figure-fitting T-shirts and jeans. To her eye, she is still too curvy, but maybe the curves don't look so bad after all.

"I start collecting compliments. They're a little bit backhanded, but they're still compliments. For example, I cannot tell you how often I've been told 'I like a woman with a little meat on her bones.' " When Victoria exercises, she tells herself that the meat on her bones is USDA choice. "I'm a little lamb chop," she jokes. "I'm a New York strip steak, with the emphasis on the strip."

When she exercises regularly, Victoria's weight hovers at the low end of her acceptable range. She may have shed only three to five pounds, but those pounds make a huge difference in her self-confidence and her sex appeal.

"I'll never look like a model," Victoria jokes, "but when I exercise I like the model that I am."

Many of us find that when we exercise, we curb our appetite. An hour on the treadmill leaves us not ravenous but sated. Exercise jump-starts our metabolism. Plus, the more we exercise, the more calories we burn when we're not exercising. A brisk walk after a heavy meal is good exercise. So is waiting an hour and then doing laps in the YWCA pool.

Eva used writing and laps to transform the self she thought of as an ungainly ugly duckling into a sleek and graceful swan.

"I wasn't about to take something like kickboxing. I wanted a form of exercise that afforded me time for meditation. Three seasons of the year, walking served me very well, but I live in a northern city, and in the winter I turned to indoor swimming. I liked it so much, it became a year-round activity for me. I'm a writer and I swear that each stroke equals the stroke of a pen. I have never written as frequently or as fluidly as I have since adding exercise to my diet regimen."

Most of us, if not all of us, are too sedentary. Unless we make a point of exercise, we do not exercise. For many of us, adding in a walk is a signifigant departure. Even twenty minutes is enough. Getting off the bus or subway two stops before our destination, taking a lunchtime stroll—these are life-affirming actions. Some people choose a more radical approach. Their daily workout may be strenuous, burning upward of five hundred calories a day.

"I can't believe it, but I'm turning into a jock," says Mary Alice, a pert blonde who always carried twenty extra pounds. "I began my weight loss with Morning Pages, which quickly told me my food was out of control. When I made my portion pie, my mandala was lopsided. I drank no water, ate no fruits or vegetables, and frequently binged on junk food. A cheeseburger and fries were my idea of a good meal, and I enjoyed them several times a week."

Mary Alice was a couch potato. She hadn't exercised in the ten years since her college crew team. While she enjoyed walking, she also enjoyed snacking while she walked. She would stop at the entrance to the park for a hot dog and soda whether she was really hungry or not. Using the four questions, she discovered that she often ate when she wasn't hungry, and she resolved to try to forge a closer link between her body and her psyche.

One evening, on an Artist Date to Barnes & Noble, she spotted a rack of exercise videos. "I'd like to look like that," she caught herself thinking, and then came the unfamiliar thought: "Maybe I can." The very next morning, just after her Morning Pages, she popped in a video. Exercising alongside the cheery instructor, she found that time sped past. "I actually enjoyed that," she thought to herself, amazed. To her astonishment, she continued to enjoy the videos. "These things are addictive," she laughed to herself. She had always been competitive, and she now enjoyed the challenge of competing with herself. An unexpected dividend reared its head: her appetite began to self-regulate. As she raised her metabolism, she actually lowered her desire to overeat. This did not show up on her scale as dropped pounds; instead, it showed up in her wardrobe as lost sizes.

"It was confusing at first," says Mary Alice. "I was losing fat and gaining muscle mass. This meant that my weight remained the same while my clothing size rapidly dropped. I invested in a good full-length mirror and several months into my regimen was shocked to find that I approved of my reflection there."

" 'You look good,' people often tell me. 'You just seem so healthy.' They don't say I look skinny, because I'm not. What I am is toned, fit, and firm. I'll take that over skinny any day."

TASK

Do You Exercise?

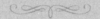

On the Writing Diet, you need to exercise to jump-start your metabolism. If you're normally sedentary, a twenty-minute walk may be enough. If you're more active, twenty minutes on the StairMaster, the stationary bike, or the treadmill may do the trick. Like Mary Alice, you may choose to exercise more—that's up to you. Pen in hand, ask yourself:

What forms of exercise do I enjoy?
What forms of exercise do I think I'd enjoy?
What forms of exercise are available to me? *— stretching + leg raises*

Even in rural areas, yoga and Pilates are starting to make inroads. You may discover there are many kinds of exercise that you do not allow yourself to enjoy. Posting at a brisk trot on a lovely horse is a potent form of exercise. So is salsa dancing. So is kickboxing. So is tae kwon do. You may find yourself saying, "I'm too old" or "too heavy" to try the form of exercise that actually appeals to you. Don't be so sure. Even in Manhattan on busy city streets one spots bicyclists in their seventies. The free-floating dance form NIA (neuromuscular integrative action) attracts people of both sexes and all ages. What you do is up to you, but do something, you must.

Pen in hand, ask yourself what exercise form would your ideal self practice? You may discover an itch to learn fencing. You might remember a love of volleyball, or a passion for touch football. Some of the fondest memories of your youth may be physical, and you may be physical still. At age sixty you might buy and enjoy a bicycle. At age seventy you might be biking still, or perhaps walking daily. Swimming is another sport that is not just for the young. Deep down, perhaps you are not the couch potato you appear to have become.

H_2O

 et us say you have been "good" on your diet and "good"
about your exercise. And the scale, the stubborn scale, refuses
to budge. What are you doing wrong? "Nothing," you answer, and
your feelings verge toward despair. There is something you are
doing wrong, and that something is so simple, it's easy to overlook.
A successful diet is one-third diet, one-third exercise, and one-third
water intake. According to nutritionist Sara Ryba, winning dieters must take in sixty-four ounces daily of pure H_2O. That's
eight eight-ounce glasses of water, more than most of us would
drink, left to our own devices.

We need to raise our consciousness about water. We need to
see it as something good and health-giving, something beneficial,
and, more exciting, something that will help us to lose weight.

"I picture myself washing the calories away," says Judy. "Every
time I eat something, I drink a tall glass of water. I picture that
water swirling through my system, washing out waste materials
and toxins."

Water does wash out waste materials and toxins. Vanity alone should be enough to start us drinking. Within a few days of high water consumption, our skin tone improves. We also seem to "wash away" any lingering bloat from our sugar consumption. Even before the needle on the scale registers a loss, we look thinner and more fit. "Have you lost weight?" we are often asked. "I'm trying," we respond. "Well, you're doing something right. You look fantastic."

Water often makes the difference between looking good and looking great. It helps us to lose pounds, but it creates an illusion of loss even before the reality.

"I hate drinking water," complains Joanie. "It just seems like make-work to me." Joanie is battling a stubborn five pounds that she could melt away using water.

"Water curbs my appetite," Fred says sensibly. "I buy bottled water by the six-pack, and keep a six-pack tucked underneath my desk. If I drink steadily throughout my workday, I have only two glasses to go by the time I head home."

"If you are stuck and the scale just won't budge, try upping your water," suggests Sara Ryba. She has often seen water "melt away" the final stubborn pounds a client is striving to lose.

"I love water," says Sonia. "I think it makes me both clearheaded and grounded. When I am in a stressful situation, I often reach for a glass of water. It is liquid clarity to me."

Michele, a judge, keeps water at the bench, where she sips at it all day. "It helps me to think clearly," Michele claims, "and it helps me to keep from gaining weight in my sedentary job."

Jacqueline, a successful dieter, orders her water by the case. "I buy some sparkling, some flat, and some flavored," she says. "When I'm bored with the water I'm drinking, I simply change styles. I write for a living, and I keep bottled water at my elbow as I sit at my desk. When I head out for my daily walk, I take water with me. I'm never far from a sip."

"I was a skeptic," says John, a lawyer who fought twenty extra pounds. "I simply didn't see how water could help me. In fact, I even thought water might be fattening, although I knew it had no calories. 'Just try it,' my nutritionist advised me. And so, because I like to think of myself as an open-minded sort, I stocked my office with water and gave my secretary the job of reminding me to drink it. 'I just hate this,' I would protest to her every time she nudged me into action, and I did hate it. But the very first week, I dropped three stubborn pounds. That was enough to convince me."

Mitchell, a hairdresser, claims that he can always tell when his clients are on a water regimen. "It shows in the skin, and a sparkle in the eyes," he asserts. "They look like they've had some work done, but it's simply water that is rejuvenating them. I've taken to drinking water myself," he chuckles.

"Water makes me feel like an athlete," says Sandy. A former marathoner, she knows whereof she speaks. "I tell myself I'm in training, that my muscles need water in order to perform. When I overdo on sugar—which I still sometimes unfortunately do—I use extra water to detox."

Successfully upping our water intake is a key to successful dieting. Some of us buy water by the case. Some of us keep it chilled in our refrigerator. Some of us make special pitchers of filtered water. We have all learned that water "works." For those who hate the taste of "plain old water," there are fruit-flavored waters and seltzer waters, which count as well. (Unfortunately, diet sodas, coffee, and caffeinated teas do not count.)

TASK

Honoring H_2O

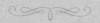

The goal is sixty-four ounces a day. Many of us fall far short of that goal. In your journal, keep a daily water log, toting up your consumption in black and white. Do you have a resistance to water consumption? Many of us do. Take pen in hand and write about your resistance. What is it about water that bothers you? Water can fill you up. When you're hit by a Snack Attack, drink a glass of water first, and then see if the hunger lingers. Often, it does not. What stratagems can you take for more water consumption? Do you need to keep water in your office? Near your television set? Near your bed? Imagine that each day is a trek through the desert. Each water break is an oasis. Plan your consumption. Give it a few days, and then step on the scale. Are those stubborn pounds slowly melting away? They often are.

Fresh Foods

*T*onight for dinner I grilled some lean turkey sausage and ate it with a chilled sliced pear. The sausage was succulent. The pear was delicious, dripping juice. The meal was so simple, it delighted me. The best things in life are often simple. Learning the simple things that please us makes for an artful life.

"When I started journaling, I began recording my daily food and I discovered that nearly all of my meals were highly processed," says Angie, the mother of four. "My idea of a quick meal wasn't salad and grilled chicken. It was macaroni and cheese or tuna casserole. On the page, my food even looked fattening. I told myself I cooked for my kids, but the truth is I was making comfort foods—and I was the one I was comforting."

"Try eating fresh foods," I told Angie. "Start your day with Greek yogurt and fresh berries instead of an Egg McMuffin."

"That sounds radical," Angie said doubtfully, but she agreed to try introducing fresh foods into her diet.

"Try salads," I urged her.

"Now you're pushing me too far," she kidded back.

We live in a land of convenience stores, in a time of convenience foods. These foods are highly processed and do not contain the nutrients we need. Fresh fruits and fresh vegetables, lightly grilled lean meats and fish—these are the foods that our bodies crave once they are given the chance to acquire a taste for them. Make no mistake: for many of us, fresh food is an acquired taste.

"I always thought of salads as a lot of work," confesses Angie. "I was shocked to find I could assemble a salad in the same amount of time it took to toast myself a Pop-Tart."

A good salad involves fresh greens and about four ounces of lean protein. That protein might be grilled chicken or steak, some tuna or salmon, perhaps some cheese. It is easy to make a good salad, and our body appreciates it when we do. Instead of getting up from our meal sluggish and dull, we find ourselves feeling energized. We have refueled in a way that our body understands.

"Writing down my foods, I was able to make progress," says Angie. "I found I could make fresh foods for two out of three meals very easily. The difference showed up both in what my scale said and what my clothing told me. I very quickly had a looser waistband."

"It's going to sound dumb, it's so basic, but I bought myself a steamer," reports June, who was fighting twenty pounds of post-menopausal weight gain. "I began steaming green beans, broccoli, cauliflower, and zucchini. I added low-salt soy sauce and some grated ginger and it was delicious. I took off five pounds before I knew it."

Over spring and summer June dropped her full twenty pounds. She went from a size sixteen to a size ten. She wasn't skinny but she was trim, fit, and youthful-looking.

"I knew I had really succeeded when my friends started asking me if I'd had a face-lift," June laughs. "The funny thing is, I no longer felt I needed one."

A nutritionist of my acquaintance calls fresh foods "the fountain of youth." She advises her clients that they are going to drop not only pounds but also years. "They don't believe me," she says. "But they come to believe what their scales and their mirrors tell them."

Stick as close as you can to raw foods and you will be on the right track. Steamed is better than boiled. Broiled or grilled is better than roasted or fried. Many fruits and vegetables are delicious raw. A well-stocked refrigerator might contain a cache of chopped celery and carrots for Snack Attack noshing.

"My tastes have changed," reports Angie. "I now prefer fresh foods to comfort foods. And I definitely prefer my new figure."

TASK

Taking Stock

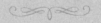

Take pen in hand. Using your journal, make an inventory of the food in your house. This means opening the pantry, cabinets, and refrigerator. Ask yourself with each item, "Is this healthy? Is this fresh? Could I substitute something better?" Most of us find we have little in the way of fresh food. We need to stock up on fresh fruits and vegetables. We have cookies and crackers, but we don't have apples and carrots. We have frozen potpies and lasagna, but we don't have quick-frozen vegetables.

"What could I learn to like?" you need to ask yourself, remembering that, yes, fresh foods are an acquired taste. Once your inventory is completed, it is time to discard the fattening foods you no longer need. Take a large cardboard carton and fill it to the brim if you can. Now is the time to discard the macaroni and cheese mix, the sugary cereals, the cheap cookies bought in bulk. Pudding mixes, canned creamed soups, tuna packed in oil instead of water, potato chips, corn chips, crackers—none of these is high in nutritive value, while all are high in calories. Canned fruits in sugar syrup, nondiet Jell-O, and, of course, ice cream and sherberts—these, too, can go. Select a friend or a charity to whom you can donate your carton of unopened foods. Take a deep breath. Change—even change for the better—can be dizzying. Take pen in hand again and write a list of healthy foods you need to shop for. List in hand, go shopping.

Sex

We live in a highly sexualized culture. Sex is used to sell clothes. Sex is used to sell cologne. Sex is used to sell beer and automobiles. Our glossy magazines are filled with images of Picture Woman and Picture Man—idealized sexualized creatures who "have it all." Did I say that Picture Woman is thin and fit? Did I say that Picture Man has a rippling torso? We are sold an image to which we aspire. That image is far thinner than the national norm. All it takes is a road trip to learn that America is overweight. Standing in line for fast food, filling up our stomachs as well as our cars at rest stations, America does not look sexy.

When we overeat, we lower our libido. We sedate our sexuality. And even if the urge to merge remains, we tell ourselves we're too plump to be pleasing.

June got divorced at age forty-five, weighing in at about one hundred forty-five. A shy woman, she turned to food for comfort in her loneliness and quickly picked up an additional ten pounds. Although she longed for companionship, she met that longing with nightly Häagen-Dazs. "Who would want me? I'm just too fat," she complained to her sisters, who were no thinner than she was but happily married. For ten years June subsisted on a diet of dreams and extra carbohydrates. While she longed to go to the movies with somebody, she settled for staying home with a video and a tube of cookie dough. When Frank asked her out, she was so startled she nearly declined. He persisted, and she accepted a dinner date.

"You know, I've wanted to get to know you for the longest time," he said, "but I didn't want to rush in."

"Ten years is a respectable grieving period," laughed June, although her ten lonely years had been no laughing matter. They enjoyed a friendly meal, and a week later, another. A month later they were still dating, and June had begun to panic about the question of bed. Frank was a charmer. He didn't pounce, but he didn't retreat either.

"You're going to say yes to me sooner or later, why not sooner?" he cajoled. Against her better judgment, June said, "All right, yes." Back in her apartment, Frank undressed her with care. "Oh," he said, "you should really wear a little sign warning people they are in for a pleasant surprise." If Frank thought June was too heavy, he didn't let on. Not that night, and not any of the many nights that followed. First they were lovers, then they became engaged, then they got married. As she became happier and less lonely, June found herself able to forgo her nightly binges.

"Food was a substitute for sex for me," June now admits. "But the substitute wasn't nearly as good as the real thing."

Like June, many of us carry extra weight that makes us reluctant to enter the bedroom. It is a vicious cycle: we eat because we miss sex; we miss sex because we eat.

Elaine, a well-to-do woman, hired both a cook and a trainer to get her into shape for a renewed sex life. She lived on a monastic diet. She underwent an Olympian regimen. She attracted the eye of Pavlo, a restaurateur. "Come eat at my place," Pavlo would coax her whenever their paths crossed. Elaine felt like saying, "I can't eat at your place, your place is too fattening! You'd never look at me twice if I made a habit of your place!" Pavlo was tenacious. Elaine was flattered and eventually accepted Pavlo's invitations, first to dinner, and then to bed.

"He tells me he likes an older woman, a woman who's experienced," Elaine says. "He tells me he likes me with a little extra meat on my bones, and I must admit, he certainly does seem to like me."

"Americans are funny!" exclaims Pavlo. "A woman is like a good steak; better if it's not too lean."

Not all of us meet Pavlos. More of us dream that a Pavlo might exist. If we are honest, many of us are overfed but starving—starved for sexuality, sensuality, and affection. If a shared meal is marked by conviviality, a binge is marked by loneliness.

"I am overweight and undersexed," says Melanie. "I have been too heavy—and too lonely—for nearly a decade. I don't like to admit it, but I have completely bought what the tabloids are selling. I am not model thin, and so I disqualify myself from any romantic encounters. When a man is interested and shows it, I think, 'There must be some mistake!' The actual mistake is my own fixation on being thin. I tell myself that when I can fit back into an eight, I can slip back into the bedroom. Right now I am a fourteen if I'm lucky."

"My body feels so plump," says Anne, "that I don't like to touch it. I can't imagine anyone else wanting to either. I know this is self-loathing, but I just can't get into those magazine articles that say 'romance yourself.' I tell myself, if I were thin, then maybe, but I am not thin. I'm twenty pounds overweight, and when I go to bed, I feel like a sack of potatoes. I don't think that's sexy, do you?"

Once upon a time, and not so long ago either, Anne's figure would have been considered ideal. A quick trip to an art museum reveals that painters such as Rubens admired a fleshy body. Flesh, however, has gone out of style. Anne is nobody's worshipped mistress.

If American reality is overweight, the American ideal is underweight. Somewhere in between lies a healthy body image that meshes with the realities of DNA and aging.

"I thought of myself as twenty pounds overweight until I asked myself what I really found attractive. It wasn't skinny, it wasn't young. It was a woman 'of a certain age' who carried curves as well as emotional ballast. This excited me. I was ten pounds, not twenty, from my goal. Ten pounds seemed doable."

TASK

What Is Your Actual Ideal?

Take pen in hand. Describe for yourself your *actual* physical ideal. Are you more rounded than rickety? Are you more sensual than skinny? Are you closer to your ideal than you had thought? If it is possible, take yourself to a large museum. People come in all shapes and sizes. Throughout the centuries, many different physiques have prevailed as icons of beauty. Allow yourself to appreciate the many different forms that have been appreciated. Are you a Rubens? A John Singer Sargent? Give yourself time to take in images of the many female forms that have inspired artists throughout the ages.

If your museum has a gift shop, buy yourself five postcards glorifying the body type that you've got. Postcards in hand, go to a café, buy yourself a cappuccino, and address the cards to yourself. Write brief affirmative messages about the beauty of your own form. You may wish to mail these cards to yourself with a simple note that says, "You're closer than you think."

Breakfast

A cup of coffee to go," we order, telling ourselves we are being smart and virtuous to begin our day by skimping on calories. But we are not being smart, and we are not being virtuous. A day that begins without breakfast begins badly. Breakfast is the fuel that powers us through our day.

"I know I am *supposed* to eat," says Carole, "but I am just not hungry. Very often it is four o'clock in the afternoon before I have found my appetite. In the meanwhile, I live on caffeine." What Carole doesn't see is that the extra weight she carries—about ten pounds—is a direct result of skimping on breakfast and then "rewarding" herself with food later in the day.

"I tell myself I've been good, and so I deserve to be just a little bit bad," laughs Carole. With the kids tumbling home from school, she makes herself peanut butter and jelly sandwiches or cookies and milk. She snacks her way through the afternoon and then eats a hefty dinner, telling herself that she deserves it since she didn't "really" eat breakfast or lunch.

The average woman requires 1900 calories per day to maintain her weight. A generous share of those calories should go toward breakfast. When we eat early in the day, we set our metabolism in motion. It burns calories quickly and efficiently as the hours tick past. When we skip breakfast, we slow our metabolism to a near standstill. Those calories we do consume later in the day burn off more slowly.

"But I hate breakfast," grouses Abigail. "There's nothing I like. I don't want oatmeal, I don't want granola. What I enjoy eating is protein, so I wait for lunch." Although Abigail likes to pretend otherwise, it's quite possible to make a high-protein breakfast. She might treat herself to lox, to grilled low-fat sausage, even to sliced sharp cheddar and an apple. Breakfast food doesn't need to be "breakfast" food.

Valerie, a vegetarian, has shaken herself loose from the tyranny of breakfast "shoulds." "I like to eat a salad for breakfast," she says. "Often I have leftover salad from the night before. It may not appeal to everybody, but for me it's the perfect start to my day."

Kiki, who loves to work out early every morning, enjoys a breakfast of yogurt with peanut butter. "It may sound awful, but it's just delicious, and it has thirty-five grams of protein. I do a lot of weight training, and I know that eating protein before and after I exercise makes my muscles respond better to the workout, and I do see the results."

For many of us, the problem with breakfast is that we are in a breakfast rut. We eat the same thing every day—yogurt with cinnamon and Splenda, for example (my favorite). We do not take the time and care to treat ourselves well. Even an egg-white omelet made with a few vegetables strikes us as too labor-intensive. Breakfast is something not to enjoy but to get over with. Once we begin to eat breakfast regularly, our appetite for breakfast increases. Keeping a food journal, we soon record if we are skimping on our early-in-the-day rations.

Of course, there are those of us who sin in the opposite direction. "I need a good breakfast," we say, and we use that phrase "good breakfast" to mean a high-calorie binge. We fix pancakes for the kids and eat just a few ourselves. We pull in at a fast food emporium and load up on eggs, sausage, muffin, and cheese, fries on the side. Telling ourselves we need "fuel"—which we do—we overfill the tank.

"I was brought up to believe in a 'good' breakfast," explains Anthony. "That meant eggs, bacon, toast, and home fries. When I tried to lose weight, I caught myself thinking, 'They *can't* mean I should skimp on breakfast!' It took real discipline to reeducate myself, to understand that yogurt and a half cup of berries, plus a cup of coffee with milk, and then a light snack would see me through until lunch. I actually found that if I ate reasonably for breakfast, I ate more reasonably throughout the day. It was like setting the governor on a car."

Using our food journal to track any resistance, most of us discover that we actually liked eating a moderate yet substantial breakfast. It does, just as we had been taught, start the day off well. When I lived in Taos, New Mexico, breakfast was the cue telling me it was time to take my dogs for a substantial walk. Loading my pack of hounds into the back of my old pickup truck, Louise, I would drive a dirt road into the sagebrush, pull over on the side, and signal the dogs that it was time for them to "go." I was signaling my metabolism the same thing. A good breakfast and a good walk both throw the switch on our metabolism to fast forward. After a lengthy loop through the sage, I would head back home to my desk and my more sedentary writer's life. The days when I skipped my morning walk, I could practically feel fat accumulating. The days when I combined a good breakfast and a good walk, I sensed my lean muscle mass.

TASK

How Do You Break Your Fast?

Take pen in hand. How do you breakfast? Do you start the day on black coffee, then treat yourself later? Do you overeat, doing your own outtake from the film *SuperSize Me*? What would you *like* to eat for breakfast? Maybe, like Valerie, you'd do best to start with a salad. Maybe, like Anthony, you need to rethink just what constitutes a good breakfast. Some of us make our breakfast treats the night before. A container of fresh fruit salad can go a long way used as a tasty garnish for low-fat Greek yogurt. Do you eat what your kids eat, telling yourself it's too much trouble to make something special for yourself? I now make a habit of checking my breakfast supplies the night before. Sometimes I need to make a late-night trip to the Korean grocer for cantaloupe or strawberries, but the outing is worth it for the morning feeling of well-being.

Refrigerator

M y refrigerator looked like a war zone, and I was the one losing the battle," jokes Dee Dee. "I kept a ready supply of high-calorie foods—jams, jellies, condiments—and very little I could actually eat. My refrigerator was my enemy, not my ally."

For many of us, our refrigerator is hostile territory. Far from being stocked with fresh and delectable foods, it becomes a catchall for leftover takeout, moldy cheeses, wilted vegetables, and spoiled fruit. We do not clean our refrigerators as often as we should, and we do not organize our refrigerators in ways that make Clean Eating likely.

"I kept a freezer full of cookies," admits Jenny. "I told myself my kids needed wholesome snacks, and that homemade cookies meant love. They also meant calories, and as I would grab a cookie here or there throughout the day, I would tell myself, 'It's just *one* little cookie.' "

Snuggled next to Jenny's cookies was a pint of vanilla Häagen-Dazs. She would often treat herself to a small scoop, never eating enough at any one sitting to set off her alarm bells. Many of us need to purge our refrigerators of high-calorie snacks. We need to learn to make smart substitutions that serve us and our families. Jenny found that her children loved fruit-juice Popsicles—low in calories and high in vitamin C. They also loved fresh fruit and squeezable yogurts. These were just as much a "treat" to them as the ice cream and cookies had ever been.

"Leftovers were my downfall," says Fred. "I would tell myself I was being wise and thrifty when I saved the remnants of a meal. What I was really doing was setting myself up with a series of high-calorie snacks." Dining out at a restaurant, Fred always took a doggie bag home, complete with the basket of uneaten dinner rolls.

"There was never quite enough for another meal, but there was always just the right amount for a high-calorie snack. I never saw this as a problem. I always thought I was being thrifty. 'Think of all the starving children in India,' my mother had taught me. I was hardly starving, but I had learned to clean my plate." A trip to Fred's refrigerator was like a stroll through a food fair. There was leftover veal Parmesan, leftover dim sum, leftover chicken curry, leftover pork satay—all of it delicious, and most of it fattening. Then, too, there was his Tupperware habit. "Whenever I cooked for myself, I saved the extra in Tupperware containers. I had Tupperware baked beans, Tupperware macaroni and cheese, Tupperware tuna salad, Tupperware chicken salad, even Tupperware strawberry-rhubarb pie."

For many of us, as for Fred, the refrigerator is a pirate's chest of culinary temptations. We keep things we shouldn't eat—telling ourselves we won't—until we do. It comes down to a handful of smoked almonds at bedtime, a slice or two of Brie on crackers, a scoop of crabmeat salad, heavy on the mayo. None of these tasty treats are real meals, we tell ourselves; they are simply snacks, but they are not the snacks we should be eating.

"I needed to rethink my entire refrigerator," says Andrea. "I sat on the kitchen floor with a big box and went through my refrigerator a shelf at a time. I couldn't believe all of the fattening foods that I was hoarding. You would think it killed me to throw away a crumb."

Like Andrea, many of us need to have a good "sit-down talk" with our refrigerator. We often find we've held on to "special occasion" foods long past the special occasion. A bottle of maraschino cherries in heavy syrup, a jar of pickled peaches, another jar of tiny cocktail franks, several containers of olives. None of these make for very legal snacking, but we tell ourselves we will "just have a bite" as we graze from item to item.

"I needed a rag, a sponge, some Fantastik, and some Clorox," Andrea reports ruefully. "While I pride myself on a clean house, my refrigerator was moldy in the corners. My vegetable drawer held wilted celery and leathery eggplant. There were droopy scallions and leeks, and potatoes sprouting eyes. I hate to admit it, but I found several frozen cockroaches. That was horrific."

Into Andrea's oversize box went jar after jar of jellies and jam, some faintly filigreed with mold. Many of the jars were long past their suggested use date. Andrea, like many of us, believed that refrigeration meant forever. For her, "fresh foods" needed an added emphasis on "fresh."

TASK

Where to Begin?

You will need a strong all-purpose cleanser, rags, sponges, a small brush, and several empty cartons. Start at the top, open your freezer door, and dig in. What's that mysterious white blob? Frozen frosting? What are you doing with three pints of half-eaten ice cream? Why does your freezer contain frozen almonds? And those quick-frozen bags of fruit are bearded with ice and look a little worse for wear. Now go to your refrigerator proper. A drawer at a time, a shelf at a time, empty your refrigerator into the cartons. Save only what is still fresh. Better yet, save only what is still fresh and still legal. Check your juice containers carefully. How many are high-calorie? You'll find most of them are. Scrub the shelves, the drawers, the door, and then situate a fresh box of baking soda within easy reach. You are now ready to re-stock your refrigerator with those items you have held on to. If you have done a thorough job, there should be plenty of room for the virtuous snacks and treats you will be buying.

Take pen in hand. Make a comprehensive list of foods you would enjoy stocking. You may find some of your choices highly personal—e.g., "a house just isn't a home without good pickles."

Using the four questions, you have by now come up with foods to eat that are legal during a Snack Attack. Be sure to stock your refrigerator fully with tempting, low-calorie options—fruits, vegetables, low-fat yogurts, diet Jell-O, and diet pudding. What you are after is the feeling of "Ah-hah! Which should I try?" Don't be surprised if you find yourself snacking less frequently—a well-stocked refrigerator leads to feelings of security. When we feel secure, we're less tempted to overeat.

Good Genes

I have a friend named Sylvia who eats whatever she wants. Grilled cheese sandwich, fries, and a malted? No problem. She stays slim as a sylph. Baklava, rugelach, strawberry cheesecake? Still no problem. Sylvia is a couch potato. She does a little yoga when the spirit moves her, which isn't very often. She's always phoning with invitations—fattening invitations. "What about some delicious dim sum in Chinatown? What about a coffee date at that terrific Italian pastry shop?" Sylvia fearlessly eats her way through Manhattan, a mecca for high-calorie dining. Eat as she does, her figure remains size four at the most. So what is her secret? Good genes.

The tabloids trail after celebrities, asking them their dietary secrets, rating their bikini bodies. Caught on the beach at Malibu, Cameron Diaz tells us she eats anything and everything she wants. What is her secret? Good genes. Movie star–good genes.

My friend Conrad, a composer, has a body composed entirely of good genes. "If you're going to write a diet book, just remember that people with good genes are sensitive. It's easy to make us feel guilty. Our friends do it all the time."

Like Sylvia, Conrad is an inveterate nosher. Cakes, cookies, cupcakes, candy—all disappear on his lanky frame. His idea of a good time usually involves dining out. "First the concert, then we'll get a bite to eat." That bite to eat is usually fattening—but not for Conrad.

Dr. Christopher Barley, my personal physician, is another well-blessed model of good genetics. At six four, he is as lean as a basketball player. I tell him that I envy his good genes. "Everybody does," Dr. Barley laughs. "But I eat carefully and get to the gym often." He sounds, just as Conrad promised, a little guilty.

Many of us grew up on the nursery rhyme about Jack Sprat and his overweight wife. Being married to someone with great genes can pose a real difficulty. Whom do you cook for? Your spouse loves the comfort of comfort foods, and they go straight to your hips. And yet, is it fair to put your lean significant other on a diet by proxy?

Vicky is five one and curvy. Every bite she eats shows on her tiny frame. For four years recently, she lived with a man graced with good genes. "He was always eating," Vicky remembers, "and he always wanted me to eat with him. At first I did, but that was a catastrophe. I had to work out for hours daily just to break even. I felt like a cotton ball, swaddled in gym clothes, always trying to work off last night's dinner. He claimed he loved me with a little extra padding, but I didn't love me. Finally we worked out a compromise—he could eat whatever his good genes allowed him; I could eat only what the nutritionist OK'd. I hate to say it, but it was a relief when we finally broke up."

The good news about good genetics, not to be catty, is that even the best metabolisms slow down eventually. "Until I was thirty-five there was absolutely no correlation between what I ate and how I looked," remembers Conrad. "I could eat anything and everything and still stay skinny. That's exactly what I did. Now that I am fifty-five I can still eat far more than other people, but I find I have a disturbing inch of pinch at my waist that I just can't seem to get rid of."

Conrad's partner laughs ruefully at Conrad's complaints. "Oh, Conrad will say, 'I think I've gained two pounds; I should lose it,' and then he continues to eat exactly the same way, but the two pounds seem to come magically off in his sleep."

If you are reading this book, you probably have at least an inch of pinch to contend with. It takes a combination of Clean Eating and exercise to bring your form into focus. Monica married a tall, thin man with good genes. To add insult to injury, he was a runner, guaranteeing that he never gained even an ounce. Although her own interests ran toward gardening, Monica decided to fight fire with fire. She acquired a treadmill, which she installed in their bedroom along with a television set. Every day while her husband gobbled his way through mountains of high-calorie food, Monica strove to eat sensibly. When he headed out the door for his run, she headed indoors to her treadmill.

"I hated that machine, but I found that with the addition of the television set, it was bearable. I worked out every morning to the morning news. Even my well-read husband soon was impressed by how well informed I was. I didn't think it was sexy, having a treadmill in the bedroom, but I felt a lot sexier when I used it."

TASK

What Are Your Assets?

Take pen in hand. Starting at the top of your head and continuing straight down to your toes, name and appreciate where you yourself have good genes. Do you have a great head of hair, beautiful eyes, good cheekbones, nice teeth? Do you have nice shoulders, shapely arms, a good bosom? Maybe you have an hourglass figure featuring a small waist. Do you have "booty" to rival Beyoncé? What about good legs, nice knees, beautiful feet, hands to match? All of us are lucky somewhere!

Pandora's Box

Many of us use food to stuff or deny our feelings. Angry with our partner, we turn to chocolate rather than a heart-to-heart. Dismayed by a child's behavior, we eat a second helping of dessert rather than set a boundary. Saddened by our aging mother's fragility, we make a large batch of buttered popcorn or turn to Oreos. We turn to food for comfort, and we turn to food for denial. "It's not really that bad," our overeating tells us as we use calories like tiny sedatives to lull ourselves into a sense of peace.

"Hell, yes, I'm afraid to diet," snaps Jennifer. "I'm hair-trigger enough. Take away my snacks and treats, and you'd have a wild woman on your hands. Who knows what kind of Pandora's box you'd be opening?"

When we alter our relationship to food, we alter our relationship to everything. Sensing this, we are often afraid to diet—afraid to rock the boat no matter how cramped and uncomfortable it may have become. Our feelings are too intense, we tell ourselves. We cannot risk unleashing them.

"There's no telling what I might do or say," says Jennifer. "I get really, really angry and I'm afraid I might say something I'd regret. Isn't it better to carry a few extra pounds and be nice?"

"Be nice" is a dictum many of us have taken too thoroughly to heart. We practice being nice rather than being authentic or honest. Our friends and families dimly sense the deception. "Tell me how you *really* feel," they may prod, but we are afraid to tell them how we really feel.

Food is the buffer we use between us and honesty. We eat the extra piece of pecan pie rather than tell our partner he leaves the kitchen a mess. "Oh, what's the big deal?" we ask ourselves as we live a tiny lie at a time. A life built on such dishonesty is a life built on mistrust. We do not trust our intimate others. We do not believe they are mature enough or strong enough to take the truth, and so we sugarcoat our dealings, falling back on Mary Poppins's adage that "a spoonful of sugar makes the medicine go down." We are often rewarded for this saccharine behavior.

"You're so sweet; you're so patient," we are told, when we are feeling anything but sweet or patient. "If only you knew," we catch ourselves thinking as we inwardly seethe with turbulent emotion. We are afraid to say how we feel. We are afraid that if we do, we will be abandoned, and so we abandon ourselves.

"My clients need to learn that unpleasant emotions are not the end of the world," explains a savvy nutritionist. "But they also need to trust that I won't give them a diet that makes them crazy with deprivation. What we are after is slow, gentle, sane weight loss. A diet of Clean Eating with sensible meals and sensible snacks actually regulates our mood swings as well."

"When I first started trying to drop weight, it was pivotal that I did Morning Pages and used my food journal," states Andrew, who often bribed himself with food when making difficult phone calls for work.

"I found I was afraid of my feelings of vulnerability. Food made me feel big and strong. I needed to learn that I could be strong without being big."

Like many of us, Andrew needed to learn that he could "feel the fear and do it anyway." In 12-step parlance, he needed to "feel everything and recover."

"It took me a while to find myself verbally, but I discovered in myself a new candor, which actually worked better than my high-powered, food-fueled sales pitches had." For many of us, Clean Eating leads the way to what might be called "clean living." When we stop using food as a sedative, we become more straightforward in our emotional exchanges. At first this may be frightening. We soon learn, however, that honesty opens the door for more honesty. Our authenticity leads to increased authenticity on the part of our spouses, siblings, and children.

"I thought my husband would kill me the first time I needed to say I was angry," relates Mary Ann. "It wasn't as bad as I thought. He looked a little startled and said, 'I didn't know you felt that way.' I was able to laugh and tell him, 'Neither did I.' "

A day at a time, a disclosure at a time, Mary Ann shared her "new" self—the self that was soon spotted in her bedroom mirror.

"It was subtle," Mary Ann explains. "It was as if each time I risked being honest I whittled away the tiniest bit of overweight. I didn't look like those before-and-after pictures in the tabloids, but I did ever so gradually start to look different. A skirt that had been too small for me suddenly fit, a blouse that had been too tight for me slid on. 'You look really nice,' my husband told me as we dressed to go out for a business dinner. 'I'll take you up on that compliment,' I flirted back. It had been years since I had made a sexual overture. Both of us were startled, but pleased."

As we open the Pandora's box of our forbidden feelings, we often move to a new level of intimacy with our significant others. Daring to reveal how we truly feel, we also dare to explore their feelings. It can be bumpy at first; it is as though we have jostled the mobile of our family dynamics. Everyone jiggles wildly before settling into a new position.

" 'This is going to take a little getting used to,' my husband told me," says Anita. "For twenty years we overate together, and when I started journaling, he felt more than a little threatened. 'What's the point of all those pages?' he would poke at me, or 'You are really going to skip dessert?' A few weeks of this and I realized that for two decades he had been my enabler, encouraging me to overeat and 'understanding' my bad feelings when I did."

"Give time time," advises a wise nutritionist. "Dieting alters the family dynamic. But the family *will* adjust."

"I was afraid I would go crazy," explains Dottie, mother of a large brood. "What I didn't expect was that I would go sane. My family was spoiled rotten. When I began to say no, they didn't like it—not at first. When I stuck to my guns, they started to respect me. It showed in the way they started to help out around the house—folding their own laundry, doing their own dishes, picking up after themselves. It doesn't sound like a lot, but it was actually a revolution. I dropped four dress sizes and traded in my martyred persona."

Many of us experience a sharp rise in our self-worth as we succeed at weight loss. Whereas we once considered ourselves "losers," we now find ourselves "winners." Afraid to face our feelings, we discover a new sense of self-confidence when we do. Opening the Pandora's box of our emotions, we discover that it is really a treasure chest holding lost talents and misplaced dreams.

TASK

Opening the Lid

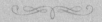

Take pen in hand. Number from one to ten. Finish the following phrase ten times, filling in the blank:

If I'd let myself admit it, I secretly feel _____ about _____.

Doing this exercise, many of us discover that we have a vast array of emotions lurking just beneath the surface. For example:

1. If I let myself admit it, I secretly feel frightened about my sister's health.
2. If I let myself admit it, I secretly feel sad about my distance from Laura.
3. If I let myself admit it, I secretly feel frustrated about my overly busy schedule.

Turn to your list and scan it carefully. With each entry, ask yourself, "Is there an action that I could take to remedy this situation?" Sometimes it is as simple as placing a long-delayed phone call. We discover that Laura is glad to hear from us. Sometimes there is no apparent action that can be taken to defuse our feelings. In those cases, we do well to practice the Serenity Prayer:

> *God, grant me the serenity to accept the things I*
>   *cannot change,*
> *The courage to change the things I can,*
> *And the wisdom to know the difference.*

We discover that if we cannot any longer medicate our turbulent feelings, we can learn to live with them. Our Pandora's box is not so dangerous after all.

The Morning After

*T*his morning I weighed myself. Just as I feared, I was up three pounds. How did that happen? I wanted to exclaim, but I knew. For the past week, despite all my knowledge, I had been backsliding. There were the four gingersnap cookies and slice of peppermint bark cake from Bunny's Bakery. There were the handfuls of cinnamon almonds. There were two luscious BLTs, and, yes, I might as well admit it, a serving of potato skins with bacon, cheese, and sour cream. You would have thought I was deliberately trying to *gain* weight, not lose it.

My Morning Pages told me clearly that I was eating to block my feelings. I was worrying about my fragile sister, who was suffering through a manic episode. I was sad that a friend of mine had undergone a botched brain surgery that left her partially paralyzed. My best friend had suffered the death of her other best friend. All of these things brought up feelings of vulnerability, sorrow, and rage. Yes, I did know what was eating me, and I was eating to medicate my feelings.

"There's nothing like a head full of AA to ruin your drinking,"

12-steppers often joke. There's nothing like a head full of diet wisdom to ruin your overeating. "I shouldn't be doing this," we think as we spoon down the Ben and Jerry's or reheat a serving of macaroni and cheese. "Something must be eating me," we speculate as we overeat. Facing it squarely, we have to admit we're in a relapse. And what are we to do about that?

"You can start over anytime," teaches nutritionist Sara Ryba. This runs counter to many of our unconscious assumptions. "What's the use?" we want to say when we have begun a binge. "I might as well just keep eating until I'm sick of it."

For years I thought I had to "finish" the binge. It never occurred to me that I could interrupt the binge, that I could stop before I literally made myself sick. Working with my food journal, I gained great insights into why and how I overate. Working with Morning Pages and the four questions, I began to become intimate with myself. I opened the Pandora's box of my forbidden feelings and found that, for the most part, I could face them after all. Then I had a week of overload, and, to my dismay, turned once again to overeating.

"What am I *doing*?" I wailed. What I was doing was self-destructing. I knew this but could not face it head-on. I rationalized. I told myself a couple of cookies couldn't really hurt. But they did hurt. I found that once I had sugar in my system, I craved more sugar. It was the same with fat and carbohydrates. I needed to get back to Clean Eating, but I wasn't sure how to do it. I placed an emergency call to Sara Ryba.

"Just start over," Ryba advised. "You don't need to 'finish' your binge, if that's what you're thinking. Turn toward water. Turn toward protein. Aim for three days of perfect Clean Eating. At first it will be hard: you will be angry; you might get headaches from sugar withdrawal. But by the third day you will feel much better, your cravings will be gone, and it will be worth it."

"Anybody can get through three days," I told myself. I took a plastic trash bag and cleaned out all of the offending foods—ice cream, almonds, cookies, cake, pie, macaroni and cheese, lasagna— from my refrigerator. I was astonished to see how many off-limit foods I had acquired in a mere week's bingeing. A trip to the grocery store, and I restocked my refrigerator with foods that were legal and appealing—fresh fruits and vegetables, low-fat cottage cheese and yogurt, quick-frozen vegetables, and for a treat, some luscious lox. I was sure to include some diet Jell-O and pudding for treats.

I needed to learn to simply get back on the horse. I needed to learn I could interrupt the self-destructive drama of a binge and return to consistency.

Rosemary, a friend of mine, tells the story of visiting a hypnotist for help with her weight. " 'You have the virgin syndrome,' he told me about my binges. 'As long as you'd gone "all the way," you needed to go even further.' I was always the one to finish the box of cookies, to eat the entire candy bar, to enjoy the final pieces of cake. That hypnotist was right. It never occurred to me that I could simply stop after a couple of cookies."

Tabloid readers have been regaled for several years now by Kirstie Alley's fight to lose weight. "I see myself as a role model for tenacity," she says. The secret of her success, she confides, is that she learned the trick of starting over rather than giving up whenever her diet became derailed.

One secret to the success of the South Beach Diet was the realism with which its founder faced relapse.

"We are human, and we are going to slip up. The South Beach Diet anticipates these slip-ups," states one practitioner. "The trick is to understand what you are doing when you binge, how it affects you, and how to get back on track as quickly as possible."

For many of us, the key to interrupting a binge lies in gentleness. Our overeating is self-destructive. Our shame around our overeating is overwhelming. We need to learn how to gently intervene on our own behalf. *for sure !!.*

"For me, the key to intervention lay in self-care," says Betty. A pretty woman, she often neglected getting manicures, pedicures, haircuts, facials, and massages. Food was her only avenue of self-nurturing, the only treat she allowed herself. Was it any wonder that she often overdid it?

"I cut my hair in a new chic style, and suddenly I was the recipient of bouquets of compliments. 'You're a handsome woman,' one man told me. I cherished that remark, and I used it as armor between me and a binge. Didn't I want to remain 'a handsome woman'? Of course I did. Recalling the compliment made it easier for me not to act out."

Margo, who belongs to a 12-step program, tells the story of attending a meeting where the topic under discussion was suicide. She was shocked by how many members told stories of actively wanting to end their lives.

"I couldn't believe the amount of self-loathing that I heard being expressed. That's when it came home to me that overeating was a self-destructive act, a slow suicide disguised as self-nurturance."

Many of us, like Margo, are loath to admit we are self-destructive. We need to face this issue squarely: overeating is an act

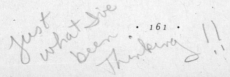
just what I've been thinking !!

yes it is!

of (self-sabotage.) Food, for many of us, is an instrument of self-loathing, not self-care.

"Every time I interrupt a binge, every time I start over, I am practicing self-love," says Dorothy, the mother of seven. "I had all-or-nothing thinking. I wanted to diet perfectly or not at all."

We do not need to diet ("perfectly.") We need to learn to forgive ourselves for a temporary relapse and start again. Each time we start, it is a victory, not a defeat. If relapse is an exercise in self-loathing, starting over is an exercise in (self-love.)

TASK

Count Your Assets

It is often difficult, on the heels of a relapse, to see and acknowledge what is good about ourselves. Take pen in hand, number from one to ten, and list ten positive ways to describe yourself. For example:

1. I am kind.
2. I am thoughtful.
3. I am funny.
4. I am enthusiastic.
5. I am thorough.
6. I am energetic.
7. I am adventurous.

8. I am loyal.
9. I am visionary.
10. I am practical.

Now take pen in hand again and, referring to your list, write out one example for each trait. For example:

1. Kind: I called my sister daily when she was sick.
2. Thoughtful: I remembered to send birthday cards and gifts to my siblings.

By counting up our positives, we are better able to combat our negatives. Focusing on our flaws and liabilities, we may feel "what's the use?" Focusing on our gifts and abilities, we may feel we are "worth" the effort of dieting.

The Magic Wand

Newcomers to 12-step recovery are often told, "I wish you a slow recovery." How passive-aggressive, they think, little realizing that a slow recovery is often a sturdy recovery. Faced with the need to lose weight, many of us are tempted by radical measures. We want the magic pill that will curb our appetite. We want the magic potion that will jolt our metabolism into fast forward. We want a liquid diet that will allow us to eliminate pesky calorie counting. The tabloids are filled with dramatic stories of sudden and extreme weight loss. Movie stars have babies, and then shed their baby weight in a scant six weeks—with the help, of course, of a strict diet and exercise regimen, usually conducted under the hawklike eyes of a personal trainer, chef, and nutritionist.

But we are not movie stars. We are real people with ordinary lives. How do ordinary people lose weight? We must find a regimen that is compatible with our daily lives, with the people, places, and events we normally encounter.

"I was a yo-yo dieter," says Marge. "I wanted to lose weight and

I wanted to lose it quickly. I brutalized my body with extreme reg-imens. Always, I saw results—a sudden weight loss followed just as surely by the regaining of every ounce I'd dropped."

Many of us, like Marge, crave a quick fix. Following the tabloids, we fail to understand that most successful weight loss is slow and steady.

When Mary Lou stopped drinking, she was twenty-five pounds overweight, bloated, and puffy. "I can't believe I let myself get in such shape," she says. But Mary Lou's shape was the least of her problems. It was far more important that as a newly sober alco-holic she maintain her sobriety rather than drop her extra pounds. "I wanted to go on an extreme diet, but my sponsor told me not to get too hungry, angry, lonely, or tired. An extreme diet was a setup, she warned me, the greased slide back to a drink." Reluc-tantly Mary Lou took her sponsor's advice. She ate three meals a day with snacks in between—particularly during happy hour, when her blood sugar dropped and she craved a drink. The first thing to go was her bloat, a residual puffiness caused by the near-lethal doses of alcohol she had been imbibing.

"You look great. What's going on with you? Have you lost weight?"

"Don't even think about losing weight for the first year," her sponsor advised, adding, "let's just get you stable." Striving to be stable, Mary Lou listened to her sponsor's advice. She began a reg-imen of cleaner eating, substituting snacks like fresh fruit or trail mix for her absent martinis. At about six months without a drink, her clothes began to fit differently. Pulling her scale from beneath the bed, where she had banished it, Mary Lou hopped on. To her delighted surprise, she was down nearly ten pounds.

"Easy does it," her sponsor counseled her when Mary Lou was tempted to accelerate her weight loss through the use of a liquid diet. "Just keep on keeping on," advised her mentor. "You're doing well so far."

And so, despite her temptation to sign on to a radical diet, Mary Lou continued to eat sensibly, now adding in some gentle aerobics. "You need the endorphins," her sponsor told her, "and exercise is an excellent time to pray."

"One day I prayed for guidance, and I heard very clearly, 'You need to write.' I began writing every morning on a regular basis. I found with the writing in place, it was far, far easier to stick to a healthy eating plan. On the nights when I was tempted to binge on Ben and Jerry's, I turned to writing instead. A day at a time, a page at a time, I began to feel more comfortable in my own skin."

A year off alcohol, Mary Lou found herself twenty pounds lighter. The change had occurred so gradually—at about half a pound a week—that she had barely noticed her own transformation.

Those of us who practice writing discover in our writing a loving witness who gently encourages us along the trail. Living—and eating—one day at a time, we often feel restless, irritable, and discontent, but these feelings pass as we stick faithfully to our regimen.

"I didn't want to hear 'Easy does it,'" protests Aaron, a highly driven type-A personality. "I wanted the drama of a sudden change. Writing about this, I discovered I was addicted to drama in all areas of my life—my work, my leisure activities, my relationships. Why should my weight loss be any different?"

"An 'Easy does it' approach *works*," Sara Ryba points out firmly.

"A pound a week of weight loss accumulates to fifty-two pounds in a year. No matter what your size, that is a substantial loss."

"I don't like to think I'm a fool," says Sally, "but I've always been fooled by the tabloid advertisements for quick weight loss. I was addicted to those bikini-clad before-and-after pictures. I looked like the before, and I wanted to look like the after. I tried fasting, potions, powders, pills—sometimes I did lose weight, but I always gained it back the moment I resumed normal eating."

What we are after is the permanent shift in lifestyle, not the quick fix of an extreme diet. If we lower our consumption by 250 calories a day and raise our exercise by 250 calories a day, that's a moderate shift that results in a pound's loss weekly. One pound doesn't sound like a lot of weight—not until you visualize a box of butter weighing one pound—*that* is the amount you have lost. A resolute dieter of our acquaintance lost forty pounds but was discouraged, feeling she still had thirty to go. "I'm not getting anywhere," she complained. I suggested that she find the concrete equivalent of forty pounds. She called us back excited. At the grocer's, she'd found two twenty-pound containers of lard. "I could barely heft them!" she exclaimed. "I couldn't believe that that was how much weight I had managed to lose. Suddenly I felt encouraged. I was more than halfway to my goal!"

Many of us, striving to practice an "Easy does it" approach, find it helpful to set goals, *modest* goals for ourselves. At one hundred seventy-five pounds, Deirdre had an ultimate goal of one hundred fifty. We encouraged her to set mini goals—five-pound increments. This meant her first goal was one hundred seventy. She reached it in five weeks.

148
5
(143) I can do that!!

"I felt like I'd broken the sound barrier," Deirdre says. "I really never thought I would weigh less than one hundred seventy again. Now I know that losing weight isn't such a mystery or something I can't do. When I control my food intake using the four questions and walk twenty minutes a day, I *do* lose a pound a week. I found I had to prove it to myself by my own experience though. If I was honest, I didn't believe that the plan would actually work for me. Now that my immediate goals are much smaller, my large goal seems attainable."

In the hyped-up world in which we live, it's hard to believe that the "Easy does it" approach could ever work. We are attracted to extremes, certain that we have to punish ourselves in order to attain weight loss. The Writing Diet, with its emphasis on Clean Eating, seems too good to be true to us. But sometimes the easy answer is the right answer.

Ted was a high-powered lawyer whose sedentary lifestyle made him prone to overweight. An athlete in his youth, he now carried an extra forty pounds. We suggested that he write every morning for a start.

"It felt very Zen to me," Ted says. "I didn't really see what writing about my life could have to do with my weight, but I began writing and soon found I was addicted to it. I was astonished by all the worries and concerns that tumbled onto the page. After a few weeks of writing, I began to feel I was a better lawyer, more focused and clearheaded. I also noticed that I had stopped 'grazing.' I got rid of the party mix I kept in my desk drawer for a quick pick-me-up. Instead, I bought apples. At the end of a month my pants were looser. I stepped on a scale and I had lost nearly five pounds."

As we raise our consciousness, we often lower our calories. Like Ted, we catch ourselves grazing on high-calorie foods. Catching on, we begin to eat differently. "Easy does it" is beginning to have its gentle way with us. At least, it will if we let it!

In the tabloids, it all happens so fast. Movie stars lose their post-baby weight in a matter of nanoseconds. They set out to be thinner, and presto! If you're Jessica Simpson, you can lose thirteen pounds in two weeks. That's thirteen pounds—or, to give you an accurate visual—thirteen boxes of butter.

"I'd love to lose thirteen pounds," says Jodi, "but I'd like to lose it instantly, just like Jessica Simpson."

Fast weight loss is a dangerous illusion. Nutritionists unite in telling us that a slow and gradual loss is more apt to be permanent.

"I like to see my clients lose one to two pounds a week," says Sara Ryba. "A slow and steady loss is more likely to be permanent."

TASK

Picture Yourself Perfect

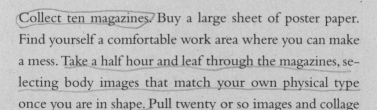

Collect ten magazines. Buy a large sheet of poster paper. Find yourself a comfortable work area where you can make a mess. Take a half hour and leaf through the magazines, selecting body images that match your own physical type once you are in shape. Pull twenty or so images and collage an idealized you. Some of us combined photos of ourselves with our ideal bodies. Many of us found that when we thought about it, we preferred a body type that was not as skinny as the tabloid norm. Like Tyra Banks, who proudly flaunts her curves at one hundred sixty-one pounds, we may exclaim, "I am still hot!"

Fit as a Fiddle

Kerry, a classical violist who has done weight training for the past three years, puts it this way: "I think people get confused by watching movie stars 'get in shape' so fast. Jessica Simpson was in terrific shape. She let her eating get a little lax, and gained some weight quickly. She pulled it together, probably eating completely clean and spending a lot of time in the gym, and returned to the body she'd had a month before. Weight that has been gained quickly can also be lost quickly, if you jump on it before it's too far out of control. Someone who's in great shape can return to that shape much more quickly than someone who's trying to get in shape for the first time."

"You mean we should go easier on ourselves?"

"I think people expect results that are unrealistic—at least in weight training, there are no quick fixes. Slowly, over years, you can build a body that is shaped exactly as you wish, and that will burn a huge amount of calories because of the high percentage of muscle mass. A person like that can get away with eating a lot of food. But the only kind of person who's going to have a six-pack in six weeks is someone who's had one before—and recently! You can't have the body of your dreams instantly, but you can feel one hundred percent better instantly after a day of Clean Eating and a good workout. Real results come slowly, but feeling better comes almost at once."

"So you're saying that we should just try one day at a time?"

"Yes, that's what I'm saying."

Kerry herself is a success story. "At my fattest," Kerry relates, "I weighed one hundred seventy-one pounds. I was drinking too much and abusing sugar. I worked out, but I would have to have trained like an Olympian to get away with what I was taking in. When I saw one hundred seventy-one on the scale and realized I weighed more than some of the men I knew, I really scared myself. I think I hit that weight for only one day, but that was one day too many.

"I began a regimen of Clean Eating, gradually cutting out alcohol and then refined sugar. I began weight training and found that working out in combination with Clean Eating was a winning ticket for me. I've lost thirty-six pounds, slowly and gradually. I'm in the best shape of my life, and I wear a size four."

Although she looks perfect to others, Kerry still has some fitness goals that she is working toward. "People ask me how I stay thin, and my first response is that that's not how I experience myself. I'm always trying to lose five pounds of love handles, always trying to increase my strength. Fitness isn't a destination; it's a daily practice that takes maintenance. When I miss a workout, I feel it. But I have made it a priority in my life, and I never stray too far off course. I certainly eat too much junk food some days, but my workouts do seem to compensate for it. And I always get right back on track after I slip up. For me, Clean Eating is a goal that I work toward daily. When I am meticulous, really eating clean and working out, I see a slow, gradual weight loss that is very gratifying."

Most of us lack Kerry's patience and persistence. These are learned traits that we, too, can acquire. The trick is not to get discouraged. Like Kerry, we may suffer setbacks, but we must learn, as she has, to "get back on the horse."

One successful dieter puts it this way: "For years I heard the phrase 'Easy does it' and took it to mean, 'Calm down.' One day I realized that the phrase actually meant 'Easy accomplishes it.' I have been successful at practicing this slogan ever since."

TASK

Easy Accomplishes It

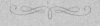

Take pen in hand. Be prepared for a little volatility. Ask yourself, what are your true feelings toward a slow and easy weight-loss program? The very concept may make you quite angry. You may not want to put in the necessary time and effort. Perhaps you're still looking for the magic wand that will render you instantly slender. What may be eating you most of all is your own impatience. That, and our many niggling worries.

For many of us, worry translates directly into weight.

Rather than act on our worries, we act out on them. Rather than using our anxiety as fuel, we use food to block our anxiety. Take pen in hand again. Number from one to five. List five current areas of worry. Now go back through your list. Next to each worry, devise one small, positive concrete action that you can take to alleviate that worry. Now do it. Remember, too, that a timely Culinary Artist Date can go a long way toward making our lives feel more livable.

One Day at a Time

*F*ood equals love. It is the most primal gesture of nurturing that we receive. As children, we yearn for the comfort of the overflowing breast. As adults, we still yearn for the sense of safety that mother's milk provided. When we are tired, when we are angry, when we are lonely, when we are fretful, we crave the comfort of food, the comfort of eating. When we feel deprived, as we so often do in our busy, hectic lives, it is to food that we turn to be soothed, comforted, and nurtured. Food makes us feel protected, food makes us feel safe. Is it any wonder that, driven by our feelings of vulnerability, some of us overeat to seek solace?

"Food is my medicine," says Anna. "When I am lonely or frightened, which is more often than I care to admit, I turn to food. In the long run, I hate the weight gain, but in the short run, I am grateful for the sense of comfort. I'm twenty pounds overweight, and every ounce was a medication I prescribed for myself."

When we begin, many of us are startled to face our fearful selves on the page. We are afraid of so many things—so much of the world seems frightening. Pen in hand, we slowly deconstruct our demons, learning to live with them one day at a time. If we take our life in daily increments, we often find we can face our fears successfully. Armed with our journal and the four questions, we are often able to eat clean in situations that once would have invited a binge.

"I have to take my overeating one day at a time," says Eleanor. "I feel like I have my finger in the dyke. I can't keep it there forever, but I can keep it there just for a day."

For most of us, success comes in tiny increments. Sweeping declarations and grandiose commitments get us nowhere. We must learn to take our cue from 12-step programs, where people pledge abstinence one day at a time.

"I remember when I first stopped overeating," says Heidi. "I had one day of Clean Eating, and I thought to myself, 'Maybe I can swing it again tomorrow.' I went to bed with a creeping sense of self-satisfaction, and even hope. When I woke the next day, I recommitted to getting one more day of Clean Eating. When I got that day, I tried for a third, then a fourth, then a fifth, then a sixth—you get the picture. One day at a time I have been eating clean for years now."

Sometimes, even a day's march seems too long for us. We reach happy hour, our blood sugar drops, and we are suddenly beset by cravings. We feel we could eat anything and everything set before us. This is when it pays to be well prepared.

"I keep a supply of ready protein," explains Adele. "Happy hour was always my downfall. Not any longer. Now I eat a couple of ounces of protein midafternoon, daily. It might be tuna fish. It might be turkey pastrami. It might be a lean sausage link. I aim at keeping my snack calories under two hundred, and I find there are so many options that I needn't panic."

Not all of us would use the word "panic" to describe our frightened feelings. For some of us, the feeling appears to be grief; for others, irritability, restlessness, or anger. At bottom, it is a feeling of dis-ease. We don't feel good in our skin, we don't feel comfortable in our bodies.

"I thought I would crawl up the walls," says Carla, who characterized herself as a "grazer," used to nibbling all day. "I tried going to a 12-step group, Gray Sheet, but their food plan seemed too extreme to me—three meals with nothing in between. I decided I might do better if I chose something less rigid."

Pen in hand, Carla devised a personal plan for Clean Eating. It included three meals a day and two snacks. This was enough food, at frequent enough intervals, for Carla to feel less frightened.

One day at a time, most of us find we can succeed. Often, what we crave as much as food is a sense of structure and safety. We may not be able to imagine going "forever" on a sensible eating plan, but we can manage to go just as far as our next scheduled food.

"I was like a baby," relates Carla. "I needed a regular feeding schedule. When I had that schedule in place and had lived with it for a while, I felt far safer."

Nutritionist Sara Ryba explains that the most difficult part of a diet is the very beginning, before we sense the safety of structure. "The first few days can be very uncomfortable," she says, and she points her clients toward the intake of extra water to soothe their cravings. "It takes three or four days to level out and get centered," Ryba explains. "But I can promise you new bursts of energy and clarity once you are through the gate."

Ryba's words are as soothing as oil on troubled waters—and some of us really need to hear them. Take Jane, a discouraged dieter.

"I complained to my therapist about my weight, and he told me that I very well might have to face it that I needed to be on a diet for the rest of my life," moaned Jane. "I wanted to shoot him. A lifelong diet? I just couldn't face it."

Fortunately for Jane, she doesn't need to face the prospect of a lifelong diet. Instead, she can try facing a diet one day at a time. Any of us can manage just one day of Clean Eating. That's three meals and two snacks. Anyone can swing it.

"Julia, you're trying to trick me with this one-day-at-a-time routine," accused Jane.

"Yes," I said. "I am."

Most of us get discouraged when we try to look at the big picture. This is why it pays to look at the small picture. It pays to ask ourselves, "How am I doing today—just today?" The answer is often, "Very well, thank you."

Our lives are built of days. Each day, well lived, builds upon the next. Starting with the daily routine of Morning Pages, we begin to view life in daily increments. "What can I do today, just today?" we ask ourselves. The answer is that we can try for a day of Clean Eating. We can manage to construct three healthy meals and two good-for-us light snacks.

"I don't know when it happened or how it happened," says Anthony, "but when I began to focus on one day at a time, my life started to be far more fulfilling. I stopped putting things off. I started really living in the now. My food changed but really my whole life changed. I began to pack more living into each day's passage. I began to treat myself better—'just for today.' "

Just for today we can manage to eat well. Just for today we can manage some exercise. Just for today we can sandwich in a little spiritual reading. . . . At day's end, instead of a to do list, we have what might be called a "ta dah" list—a sizable handful of things well done. We couldn't face the prospect of being so virtuous for the rest of our lives, but a day at a time, it's quite possible—even enjoyable.

"A day at a time, I have now built up years of abstinence from bulimia," says Gayle. "I couldn't face the idea of the rest of my life, but a day at a time, that's precisely how it is turning out, and I am so glad."

" 'You're so productive!' people often exclaim to me," says Diana, a successful television writer. "I sometimes try to tell them that it is because I live one day at a time, but when I say that, their eyes glaze over. They think there has to be some other secret that I am not telling them. I tell them there is one big secret, 'One day at a time.' That's the secret to my prolific writing career. That's the secret to my long-term relationship. It's even the secret to how I walk my dogs."

A day at a time, we not only diet, we live. We undertake marriage. We go back to law school. We write books. We do many things and we do them very well because we are doing them in tiny increments not in large, overwhelming bites.

TASK

One Day at a Time

Take pen to page. Ask yourself what commitments you can make "just for today." You may find that when you ask this question, your mind skitters a bit in panic. "Sure I can do this for today, but what about tomorrow?" you may catch yourself thinking. Don't think about tomorrow. Tomorrow can take care of itself tomorrow. Just for today, what is possible?

Eating to Please

The crowd is festive and the restaurant is chic. The revelers sit elbow to elbow at a large table. Pitchers of sangria invite participation. "Will you have a little?" I am asked. I decline the wine but reach nervously for the bread basket. I am on a no-carbohydrate regimen, but that fact fades from consciousness as I butter a slice of bread. Bad enough that I don't drink, but if I don't eat, too, that's a party spoiler, or so I tell myself.

The restaurant is chic, the crowd is more chic. I want to fit in. A decision is made to order family style. This means that both appetizer and entrée will be chosen for me. I hear the mention of fried plantains, not a staple on my diet. Also, sausages, guacamole, empanadas, and more bread. A diner grasps me by the arm. "Julia, for a moment there I thought you were drinking," she says. "No, no," I assure her, and point to my empty water glass. "I'm so relieved," the diner breathes. "I know you're sober a long time, and I'm eight years without a drink now myself." "No, no drinking tonight," I assure her. I don't say what I'm thinking: How can I possibly get through this meal without overeating?

The guest of honor sits directly to my right. She has chosen the restaurant with care, selecting a festive cuisine to please her party. I do not say to her, "Natalie, this food is off-limits for me." Instead, when the food is passed, I load my plate and then pick at the delicacies I've been offered. I should be stronger, I tell myself. I really shouldn't eat these things. But I do eat them, and I eat them because I am eating to please.

Many of us eat to please—not ourselves, but our significant others. Left to our own devices, we might do quite well; bypassing the bread basket, skipping dessert. Eating with others, it seems rude to say "no thank you." It is also embarrassing, as if we had taken a black Magic Marker and underlined the fact that we are overweight.

For five years now Lorna has dated Daniel. Daniel is tall and slender, a hearty eater blessed with good genes. Lorna is tall but not so slender. What she eats—or doesn't eat—shows.

"I'm a yo-yo dieter," Lorna says woefully. She and Daniel live in separate cities. When he comes to stay with her, she cooks luscious meals for him, often joining him in a celebratory glass of wine and a delectable dessert. The pounds pile on. Every time Daniel comes to visit, Lorna gains between five and ten pounds. She sheds them again as soon as she is on her own. "Without Daniel I don't drink and I don't eat sweets," Lorna tells me. "When I'm with him I eat what he wants to eat, not what I do."

Lorna, like so many of us, believes that food is love. She shows her love for Daniel by joining him in extravagant meals. She is afraid to diet in his presence for fear he will find her a wet blanket. With her lighthearted temperament and ready humor, Lorna is anything but a wet blanket. What she lacks is not humor, but adequate self-love. Although ostensibly an independent woman, she is secretly clingy. Her codependence shows when it comes to food.

Working with your journal, you can anticipate some of the meals at which you will be tempted to overeat to please. Holidays and special occasions invite dietary abuses. Pen in hand, you can plan your indulgences, planning, too, ways in which you can curb your calories. At Thanksgiving you might tell yourself "a little dab of everything, but no seconds." When the pressure is on, it may be a good idea to place before and after calls to our Body Buddy as well. I should have done this with the fête at the restaurant.

"An ounce of prevention is worth a pound of cure," the saying goes, and we can prevent our overeating through journaling, communicating with our Body Buddy, and through prayer—yes, prayer. Seated by the dinner rolls, we can pray, "Dear God, please help me." Then we can pass the rolls farther along the table and sip at our water. Of course, there are some people who will notice our abstinence and not approve. "Aren't you going to have at least one roll? They're delicious," we may be prodded. It is sufficient to simply say, "No, thank you," and change the subject. This is often enough. When it is not, we need to remind ourselves that other people, too, can suffer from a toxic relationship to food. Your cousin Mary Beth may want you to have a dinner roll so that she herself can have two. Very often our weight problem is invisible to any eyes but our own.

"You look beautiful, Julia," I was often told as my weight teetered at a new and dangerous high. Weight control, ideally, is a matter of autonomy. We eat for ourselves, for our own tastes and needs, and not for the agendas of others. Yet others often offer their opinions.

"You must try some of your aunt Helen's cheesecake," we may be told. "You must try your aunt Minnie's crumb pie." And so, against our best resolutions, we often find ourselves weakening. "I'll have just a sliver," we say. "I'll take a tiny piece." Yesterday's sliver and today's tiny piece may go straight to our waistline or contribute to tomorrow's cellulite bloat. "I was doing so well!" we may moan, finding ourselves, like Lorna, giving in to our need to please.

TASK

Pleasing Ourselves

Take pen to page. Write out the worst scenario you can imagine if you refuse a dining experience. Let us say you do not eat Aunt Minnie's crumb pie. Will Aunt Minnie wail, cry, shoot you? Give your imagination free rein. Allow humor to enter the picture. What, precisely, do you expect to happen if you stand up for yourself? Allow yourself to write a triumphant scenario in which you successfully decline food you do not want or need. Imagine yourself stepping on the scale post-holiday to discover not an extra five pounds but steady as she goes. How would it feel to stick to your own agenda, and even lose weight during the holiday season? It's possible.

Lingerie

I try to think of myself as a Christmas package," says Rita. "I want to be wrapped as prettily as possible." Rita is a large woman who is using the Writing Diet to become smaller, but she has decided to not defer her sexuality until she is slim.

"I think red is sexy," says Rita. "I wear as much red lingerie as I can find. I like it because even though it doesn't show and no one knows I'm wearing it, I still know. I think of it as a small flag of my sexual nature."

Unlike Rita, many overweight people place their sexuality on hold "until. . . ." We wear styleless lingerie, underwear in drab colors that serve only to underscore our sense that we are lacking in appeal.

"Face it," says Anne, "fat isn't sexy." And so, to prove her point, she wears what she laughingly calls industrial strength underwear. There's nothing attractive about it. She wouldn't want to be seen in it. But she tells herself her odds of being seen in it are very slight.

Dolores has a very different attitude. Her lingerie is always pretty and feminine no matter what her size. "I enjoy it," says Dolores, "and I think my lovers do too." Dolores works daily with the positive affirmation "I am sensual and sexual." Is it any wonder she attracts suitors? "I think of my lingerie as a sign of my self-worth," she explains. "I had to learn to let myself be pretty."

Many of us can take a leaf from Dolores's book. We, too, need to learn to be pretty. We may find we fit the larger sizes from Victoria's Secret. Or we may find we need to buy "sensible" underwear and then use Rit dye to transform plain white into something lovelier.

"I told myself I'd wait to be thin before getting into bed with anyone," says Anita. "But that was before I met Jim. He seemed to like me just as I was, and so I went lingerie shopping so we'd both like me when I took my clothes off."

Caroline believes it's a case of "act as if." "I was brought up a good Catholic girl with good Catholic underwear," she says. "I had to learn to be sensual. I had to learn to dress the part."

Dorothy, as the mother of a large brood, always deferred shopping for herself. "They need the treats more than I do," she reasoned. But I urged her to find time and money for herself. "I feel like a girl," she reported back. "Nice lingerie seems so frivolous and decadent. I can't believe it's mine, but I love it." As a footnote, Dorothy blushingly adds that her husband has noticed her new finery and seems to find it "attractive."

Many of us have to get over a "martyred" mode of dressing. Overweight and oversize, we tend to think of ourselves as draft horses—good workers but little else. It is a shock to find that we are still sexually appealing. Not all men are attracted to skinny women.

"I like a woman with a little flesh on her bones," remarks Anthony.

"Who wants to make love to a stick?" asks George.

Dressed in feminine finery, we send a signal—to ourselves first and then to others—that we are lovable, sensual, and sexual.

"I always skimped on underwear," says Jenny. "I figured no one sees it, so, so what? It took a real effort for me to spend money on intimate apparel. I was shocked at how much better it made me feel once I had."

"Out of sight, out of mind" is the attitude many of us take toward lingerie. Little do we realize we take the same attitude toward our sexuality. Waiting to be thin to be sensual, we often cause ourselves a low-grade depression. We need to be touched. We need a physical expression for our affections, but we deny ourselves this right.

"I was embarrassed to go shopping for lingerie," says Elizabeth. "I simply did not want to face myself in a department store mirror. For a long time this meant I did no shopping. My lingerie was in tatters before I thought to turn to the Internet. With a little searching, I located a treasure trove of larger-size lingerie. When my packages came, I felt like it was Christmas. I tossed out all of my 'low self-worth' belongings and really let myself enjoy my new 'luxuries.' They made me feel so much better, I soon concluded they weren't luxuries at all."

Sometimes a little lace can go a long way toward curing low self-worth. A shot of color can be a real shot in the arm. A floral pattern might remind us we are the bloom that needs tending to. Spritely stripes and polka dots bring with them good humor.

It's hard to be depressed when you wake up in the morning and put on good lingerie. It's hard to feel you're going to have a terrible day when it starts off so nicely.

There is a lingerie ad with the slogan "Sometimes a woman deserves a little unfair advantage." I have learned that "sometimes" means "always."

TASK

Treat Yourself Well

Go to your lingerie drawer. Sort and discard any and all "low self-worth" lingerie. Now take yourself shopping. Let yourself purchase at least one beautiful bra and some pretty panties. Remember that money thus spent is money well spent, and allow yourself to splurge just a little.

If this exercise strikes you as particularly difficult or undoable, take pen in hand. Number from one to five. Finish the following phrase:

The reason I can't have lovely lingerie is . . .

You may discover age-old conditioning that still dictates your behaviors. Provoke your subconscious onto the page,

where you can grapple with it in the open air. Now take
pen to page and number from one to five again. Complete
the following phrase:

If I had nice lingerie, I'd ... be sexy

Often we are afraid of setting a "wild woman" loose.
Most of us can afford to be a little wilder than we are.

Trauma

Many of us carry extra weight defensively. Our weight is a buffer intended to protect us from real or imagined harm. Sometimes our weight is a reaction to an actual harm from our past. At other times it is the barrier we construct to protect ourselves from harm in our future. One thing is true in all cases: although we intend our weight as a weapon against others, it boomerangs back onto ourselves.

This was the case with Gretchen, the victim of a violent rape during her late teens. She told no one of the attack, and she told herself that she was strong enough to get over it. Faced with terrible feelings of vulnerability, she barricaded herself behind an ever-escalating amount of excess weight. By the time she reached her mid-thirties, when I met her as a creativity student, she wore an extra hundred pounds as armor. From the front of the classroom I quickly saw the fragility she masked with anger and overweight. "Write," I told her.

Although it frightened her to do so, a day at a time, a page at a time, Gretchen began to write. It wasn't too long before the painful memories of her attack surfaced in her daily Morning Pages. "I'm scared! I'm angry! I can't face all this!" she protested. I urged her to keep writing when she felt like stopping, and almost against her better judgment, she did. As she wrote, her volatile feelings became less volatile. Telling herself her story, she felt the stirrings of compassion. She faced, even tamed, her demons. One dramatic evening she shared her story with the rest of the class, ending by saying, "I realize now I no longer need to be fat to defend myself." In the weeks that remained, Gretchen's weight began slowly to drop off. She was writing her way into a state of health.

"I've always dreamed of being a playwright," Molly, an overweight woman in her mid-fifties told me. "The problem is, I'm afraid to write. Have you ever had anyone go crazy?"

I assured Molly that I had never known writing to drive anyone crazy, but I said to her, "Try writing, and if issues surface that feel traumatic, promise me you'll get help." Molly began writing. Three weeks into Morning Pages, she had a breakthrough and wrote her first short story. This was the good news. The bad news was that the story's subject matter was incest. Reading the story, I asked Molly whether she had any blocked memories from her past.

"I think so," Molly said tentatively. "I've always wondered. Do you think I should get some therapy?"

"Yes," I suggested, "I think you should." And so, while continuing to write her Morning Pages, Molly undertook an incest recovery program. As her memories surfaced, she was able to release them safely in a therapeutic setting—but her memories weren't all that surfaced. Her long-delayed dream of playwriting emerged with an increasing sense of urgency. Scared to try but scared not to, Molly undertook writing her first play. Week by week she worked at her craft. From the front of the classroom I could see her changing from a timid, pudgy woman to a more slender and confident one. Class ended with Molly safely launched into both writing and weight loss. It was six months later that I opened my mailbox and received a catch-up note from Molly.

"I thought you would like to know that I won my first play-writing contest," she wrote. I felt both proud and gleeful for her.

If pounds are the barricade we put between us and trauma, words are the chisels with which we take our barricades down. Writing about our injuries and injustices helps us to make peace with them. As we forgive and let go of our past traumas, we move toward brighter and more hopeful futures.

"I came from a violent home," says Lorna, a tall, lovely, but overweight woman. "I tried to put all that behind me, but I simply stuffed my feelings with food. When I undertook Morning Pages, I knew that my past would resurface—and it did. A day at a time, a page at a time, I found myself facing my terrible memories. Unexpectedly, I felt compassion, not only for myself but for my troubled father. He, too, had come from a violent home, and was doing the best he could to raise us."

Not surprisingly, Lorna had repressed feelings of anger as well as vulnerability. This is true for most of us with buried traumas. It often takes a bit of sleuthing to uncover our own volatility as well as vulnerability. Lorna worked with the phrase "If I let myself admit it, I feel angry that . . ." To her shock and surprise, she had more than fifty entries in this spot-check inventory. She was angry about many things, large and small. Although she never thought of herself as an angry woman, she clearly was one. From the front of the classroom I watched Lorna's progress a week at a time.

"I feel stuck," Lorna told me, but she was stuck no longer. A page at a time and a pound at a time, her angers began to dissolve. "I don't know who I am!" she exclaimed to me one evening. I could understand her confusion. To my observer's eye, she had lost several dress sizes. Additionally, she had signed up for ballroom dancing—a long-deferred foray into a lighthearted and flirtatious world.

Another student, Mary Elizabeth, experienced misplaced feelings of terror that she tried to block with food. As the pounds escalated, so did her fears. When she began creative recovery, she was nearly agoraphobic—frightened to venture into what she feared was an unfriendly world.

"I don't know what it is with me," Mary Elizabeth complained.

A month into Morning Pages, she did know what it was. Memories of sexual advances by her older stepbrother surged into mind.

"I thought I had dealt with Billy and the fact that he was a bully. But he was worse than a bully—he was a predator."

"Not all the world is predatory," I assured Mary Elizabeth. In her Morning Pages and on her Artist Dates, she was discovering a benevolent, hitherto unexplored world. "I'm starting to feel some optimism," she reported to me.

"You may still need some therapy," I advised.

Open-minded and brave, Mary Elizabeth undertook therapy with an innovative therapist who saw the value of writing as a therapeutic tool.

"I'm getting lighter and lighter-hearted" was Mary Elizabeth's last report to me. She had channeled her abundant creativity into the writing of children's books.

"I love what I'm doing," she told me.

For many of us, Morning Pages hold the key to shifting our lives from reactive to active. No longer the passive victims of unwanted trauma, we find ourselves able to create healthy scenarios within our own lives. Is it any wonder we become slimmer as our need for armor slips away?

TASK

Writing Things Right

Set up a safe and nurturing environment for yourself—a familiar chair, some soothing music. Now take pen in hand and gently scan your own psyche. Finish this phrase, "If I let myself admit it, I feel traumatized that_____." Use the phrase ten times. All sorts of unexpected answers may spring to mind. "I feel traumatized that I was sent away to boarding school." "I feel traumatized by Dan's date rape my senior year." "I feel traumatized that my mother had twins and had no more time for me."

Even if you consider yourself to be quite well adjusted, don't be surprised if you are able to come up with a list of traumas. If you find the word "trauma" overly dramatic, try using a milder phrase. "It still bothers me that_____." Your list may turn out to be longer than you think.

You may feel a little like the princess in "The Princess and the Pea," traumatized and bothered by seemingly small

I didn't or don't have clarity

occurrences. You still smart over grammar school slights. What Sister Ann Rite said to you in fourth grade is still eating at you—and you are eating at it. The act of moving a trauma from your subconscious to your conscious mind is very healing. You'll notice an increase in your emotional palette. You'll have access to feelings you have long overlooked. You are more colorful than you have previously imagined.

Clothes

"Clothes make the man," runs the old adage, but we like to think we are above all that. Telling ourselves that clothes don't matter, we slowly and gradually suffer from a shrinking wardrobe as fewer and fewer of our clothes fit us any longer. Perhaps we used to be a size eight and we are now a size fourteen. That's not so "fat," but it's fat enough that our size eight clothes no longer fit.

Discouraged and dejected, we are afraid to go out shopping. We don't want to invest in larger-size clothing. We don't want to face the cruel reality of department store mirrors.

"I hadn't really shopped in three years," relates Andrea, a kindergarten teacher. "I had a few shapeless black outfits that I told myself made me look thinner. I wore them week in and week out. I love gay colors but they were history for me. I dressed like the Wicked Witch from *The Wizard of Oz*. My poor children!"

When Andrea told me her story, I heard a tale of decimated femininity. Her shapeless black outfits were harsh and unflattering. They were depressing and, yes, Andrea was depressed. I urged her to try a shopping trip. Even one outfit would be a breakthrough. It took a little coaxing, but finally Andrea decided to try.

"I found a beautiful tawny skirt-and-tunic ensemble," Andrea reported. "I couldn't believe that it fit me and that I could afford it. When I wore it to school, the kids were in shock. So were my colleagues. One teacher asked me if I had fallen in love!"

We do need to fall in love—with ourselves. We need to dress ourselves in attractive and appealing clothing, the kind we might wear if we did have a new beau. Instead of suffering through a regimen of basic black, we need to choose colors that flatter us. We need to shop for apparel in sizes that actually fit.

Janet lived in a chic New York neighborhood that was filled with adorable boutiques holding clothes that were too small for her. "I felt like the Incredible Hulk whenever I set foot in one," she recalls. "Nothing fit me and I felt like I could sense the salesladies' contempt."

I suggested to Janet that she try a shop that specialized in larger sizes. She recoiled in horror. "I am not that fat," she snapped. Perhaps not, but she might enjoy the experience of shopping where her size is not an issue, I told her. Angrily and reluctantly she decided to follow my advice.

"You won't believe the outfits I scored!" she later all but hooted in triumph. "I got skirts, tops, slacks, something to wear to the country club dinner dance! I am a new woman—thank you!"

It doesn't take a lot to make a large difference. If your wardrobe has dwindled down to the one or two outfits that you live in, then one or two new outfits will double your wearable clothes. Realizing this, Isadora decided to dust off her childhood 4H sewing skills.

"I had a wonderful time fabric shopping and it took me only an afternoon to run up my first outfit," gushes Isadora. "It was pretty. It was flattering. It was inexpensive compared to store-bought clothes. I felt like I had just been let out of jail. I made myself two more outfits in rapid succession and I felt like a fashion plate. Not to mention how much fun I had. I'd forgotten how much I love to sew."

Not all of us can sew and not all of us would wish to. Another option is to seek out the help of a good seamstress. Often a tailor-made dress costs less than its store-bought counterpart. Often it is far more flattering, as you can choose your own fabrics and colors.

"It doesn't sound like much," relates Andrea, "but I had a dress made up for me in navy blue. It was still dark. It was still flattering, but it wasn't black, and that made all the difference."

A good seamstress is smart about figure-flattering styles. She may suggest that you show off a small waist or a fine bustline. If you are accustomed to shapeless smocks, a well-tailored dress can be a shock to the system. You may still be overweight, but you don't feel sexless and unattractive. You look womanly, and that has appeal.

"Dress the part," we are told, and it pays to think about this advice a little. Just what part are we dressed to play? Wife? Mother? Lover? Worker? Dressed in our low-self-worth apparel, we are often dressed as martyrs. Our clothes signal our poor self-image and people may unconsciously treat us accordingly. Rather than dressing for success, we have unwittingly dressed for failure.

"With all my drab and shapeless black, I looked like something out of *Marat/Sade*," exclaims Andrea. "My clothes practically shrieked, 'Use me! Abuse me!' And people did."

"But, Julia, isn't transformation supposed to be an inside job?" I am sometimes asked.

Yes and no. Change begins on an interior level, but as we work on ourselves, we begin to make different choices. We can choose to show ourselves. We no longer need to dress to hide. Like a loving parent with a neglected child, we often find that a special outfit signals "I love you." That message registers first with ourselves and then with the world at large.

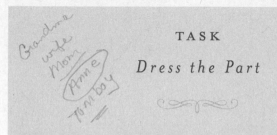

TASK

Dress the Part

Settle into a comfortable chair. Take pen in hand. Ask yourself, "What parts do I play? Do I have clothes appropriate to my parts?" Jot down your roles. Jot down the clothes you have that fit those roles. You may write down "lover" but have no romantic outfit in which to play the part. You may write down "teacher" but not have anything crisp and tailored. You may have "mother" clothes but no "sports" apparel. You may have one outfit that you wear role to role to role.

Now open your closet. Make a written inventory of its contents. Are there clothes you have forgotten about that could be pressed into service with a little alteration? Waistbands can often be expanded by an inch or two. Seams can be let out to accommodate your new, more ample hips. Sometimes you are merely missing a button or a hook and eye. Make a stack of mending. Make a stack of those items needing alterations. Make a list of items that are truly missing and will need to be shopped for.

Make yourself a cup of tea. Job well done.

Mirrors

*T*o most dieters, mirrors are no laughing matter. But Lisa likes to make a joke: "Mirror, mirror, on the wall, who's the scariest of them all?" Like many of us, Lisa believes that there are "good" mirrors and "bad" mirrors, and that "bad" mirrors can be downright frightening.

"When I started, I was twenty pounds overweight. That's what my scale told me, that's what my common sense told me, that's what my nutritionist told me. My scary mirror told me something else. I wasn't just overweight—I was grotesquely obese. I was ugly, awful, a monster. Every time I looked in that mirror I saw and believed the worst. Dieting was impossible for me; I was simply too far gone."

When Lisa told me about her scary mirror, I suggested she get rid of it. This struck her as heresy. Wasn't her mirror like a tough-love friend? Didn't she need to know "the truth"? I explained to her that there really were good mirrors and bad mirrors, and that using a bad mirror was not in her own self-interest. Still, Lisa found it difficult to simply throw the mirror away. I suggested she set it in the lobby of her apartment building to be claimed by someone else.

"Use at your own risk," Lisa scrawled on the note that she left with the mirror. Then she went out hunting for a "good" mirror, and was surprised to find one she could readily afford. "My good mirror is optimistic," Lisa says. "I look just a little better than I actually think I do, and that gives me the incentive to diet, since I'd like to look better yet."

Some diet Nazis might say that a good mirror is "cheating." I would say a good mirror is encouraging, giving us a glimpse of our future, if we just stick to our guns.

Like Lisa, for a long time Maggie lived with a "bad" mirror. It had one of those funny ripples, and that ripple hit just at Maggie's hipline, where she had ripples herself. As she assessed herself in her bad mirror, Maggie's figure was always hopeless. No outfit looked good on her. No outfit was slimming. Sometimes Maggie went straight from her mirror to her refrigerator, figuring, "Oh, what's the use?" Like Lisa, Maggie needed a new mirror in order to see herself with forward-looking eyes. Unlike Lisa, Maggie couldn't quite muster the strength to simply pitch her offending mirror. Fortunately she made an appointment to have her apartment painted, and one of the painters shattered her mirror. Maggie was astonished at how much better she felt living without it. When the painter offered to replace it, she nearly declined. Then she thought, "Maybe Julia's right, and it was a bad mirror. Maybe I can look for a good mirror in its place."

Good mirrors are surprisingly easy to find. Most hardware

stores carry full-length mirrors, and a quick glimpse is all it takes to tell you whether the mirror is friend or foe.

It took Maggie three hardware stores before she found mirrors that felt friendly. When she did, she bought two of them—one for her dressing area and one for the foyer for a last-minute check before she stepped from the house.

"Having a good mirror is a real ally. I'm still too hippy, but I'm not grotesque. And as I have lost a few pounds, my mirrors have become even friendlier."

Some of us have tried living without any mirrors at all. For most of us, this takes just a little more faith than we can muster. Like living without a scale, life without a mirror can seem a little too radical. Just as the scale gives us a rough idea of our actual weight, a mirror gives us a rough idea of our actual image, and that image is changing. Lisa found that once she got rid of her unfriendly mirror, she spent more time with her friendly mirror. She began to experiment with different looks, making a shift away from the shapeless basic-black clothes that had been her staple. With the help of a tailor who came to her house and worked with her in front of her friendly mirror, Lisa crafted several figure-flattering outfits. "I might still be overweight," she explained, "but I have got a small waist and with the right clothes, I can show it off." Instead of unpleasantly plump, Lisa began to see herself as curvaceous. This adjustment in attitude was a direct gift of her new mirror.

For Darlene, who had gone for many years with no mirror, the idea of finding a friendly mirror seemed threatening and difficult. I urged her to try her neighborhood hardware stores, and at the second one, she encountered a mirror she felt she could live with. "It's quite a shift, living with the feedback from my mirror," Darlene told me. "I would have said that ignorance is bliss, but now I say that knowledge is power. I know what I look like and I know what my clothes look like. It's not as bad as I feared, and not quite as good as I'd like, but I think of my mirror as a source of guidance to help me move in the right direction."

Darlene has a self-loving attitude. She embraces progress, not perfection. For her, as for many of us, a friendly mirror is a genuine ally, a loving source of self-knowledge and support.

For many of us, using a mirror regularly is like taking a healthy dose of truth serum. We see where we are and what we need to change. For some of us, our mirrors are an effective defense against the bad mirrors that we frequently encounter when we go shopping.

"What is it with retailers?" Maggie wants to know. "They'd sell a lot more clothes if their mirrors were a little kinder." True enough, but often a retail mirror is a bad mirror—one that makes even the slimmest among us feel pudgy.

Carol is a size four. To the casual eye she appears trim, even slender. In a bad mirror, however, Carol locates imaginary love handles and tells herself she needs to drop ten more pounds and two more sizes. I suggested to Carol that enough was enough, and that she try finding a household mirror that did not distort her lovely figure.

"You mean it's that simple?" Carol demanded. "I just shop for a mirror until I like what I see?"

"Yes."

TASK

Mirror, Mirror on the Wall

Most of us live with multiple mirrors—some kind, some not so kind. We may have a "good" mirror for makeup which we routinely use. Take your pen and journal in hand and move mirror to mirror within your space, carefully recording what you find in each encounter. You may discover one "good" mirror and five "bad" mirrors. You may discover five "good" mirrors and one "bad" mirror. What you are after is friendly objectivity, a mirror you can use without wincing. You may not be able to purge all of the "bad" mirrors with which you've been living. In that case, it is important that you acquire a "good" mirror. Take yourself to your local hardware store and search for a mirror that says "I like you" when you look into its depths.

Dessert

I don't mind dieting, I just hate giving up dessert," exclaims Annie—who speaks for most of us. We can face the deprivation of low carbohydrates and lean proteins. We can even learn to like Clean Eating. But can we really give up desserts? For most of us, the honest answer is no, and so we must devise an eating plan that includes dessert in some form.

If you have given up refined sugar, fruit becomes a surprisingly potent source of sweetness. You may discover that it is highly satisfying to end a meal with a cup of freshly sliced berries dusted with Splenda. Alison found that frozen berries whipped in the Cuisinart with one-third cup ricotta cheese and Splenda yielded her a delicious dessert parfait, as satisfying as a bowl of ice cream—maybe even more satisfying because there was no guilt.

Nutritionist Sara Ryba advises her clients that the initial withdrawal from sugar may take three to five rough days. "But then your tastes change," she promises. "You will no longer crave sugar as you once did."

Using our journals to explore our feelings, many of us discover there is a direct link between our feelings of loneliness and unlovability and our cravings for sugar.

"Sugar—especially chocolates—was my way of saying 'I love you' to myself," confesses Rhoda. "I didn't believe the nutritionist's promise that I would be free from cravings, but I found that after five days of Clean Eating, my tastes really did alter. Fruit became a satisfying sweet, and my food plan afforded me two full servings of fruit daily."

"I don't miss the bloat," jokes Suzanne, who looked pounds thinner a mere week into her recovery. The bloat, of course, was sugar bloat, and her combination of Clean Eating and intensive water consumption did indeed seem to magically "wash the bloat away."

"I have cheekbones!" she crowed. "And I can't wait until I have hipbones again too." To satisfy her sweet tooth, Suzanne turned to diet Jell-O and cantaloupe. To her astonishment, she did not miss her sugar highs. As for so many of us, her sugar highs had inevitably been followed by sugar lows, making her day a roller coaster of warring emotions.

One of the first results of sugar withdrawal is a more even temperament. Sugar, after all, is a stimulant, which often makes our emotions hair-trigger. The natural sugars found in fruit are far easier for our system to metabolize. We are not triggered into acting out on our emotions.

"I thought I had a problem with rage," says Bernadette. "What I really had is a problem with sugar." For Bernadette, her withdrawal from sugar brought an unexpected and welcome stability.

She no longer flew off the handle, ranting at her husband and children in "justified" tantrums.

"One woman asked me if I'd had a spiritual experience," says Bernadette. "That's when I realized how radical the change really was."

Quick-frozen fruits whipped in the blender make a creditable sorbet. As mentioned before, quick-frozen fruits plus ricotta and Splenda make a fine fake ice cream (it even contains protein as an added benefit). Fresh fruits—sliced, pared, or chopped, with a little cinnamon and Splenda—can be a real delicacy.

"I can't believe I gave up my cookie habit," Katherine told me. Her voice sounded gleeful and relieved. Most of us do feel gleeful and relieved when we discover we can live happily and healthily without refined sugar.

"I didn't just have a sweet tooth," says Mary Elizabeth, "I had a sweet fang." Journaling taught Mary Elizabeth that her sugar consumption was directly connected to her anger. "If you hurt me, I'd hurt me," she relates. A month into the Writing Diet, she found herself expressing her anger more appropriately. "I learned to say, 'Ouch, you hurt me' instead of 'Please pass the ice cream.' "

Greater emotional authenticity, greater fluidity and self-expression, increased self-confidence and self-worth—all of these are benefits of a sugar withdrawal. And did I mention weight loss? Giving up sugar jump-starts weight reduction. Life is simply sweeter without the sweets.

TASK

Your Just Desserts

Take pen in hand. Number from one to seven. Devise seven sugar-free desserts. Treat yourself to one per day in the week that follows. Note: these desserts do not need to be complicated. Use your imagination. You might want to sip a diet cream soda after your dinner. That's a dessert. You might want to "bake" an apple or a peach or a plum in the microwave. Sprinkle with Splenda and it's nearly a cobbler.

The Grace of God

I look ungodly," we often say, glimpsing ourselves in a passing
mirror, overweight and overwrought.

"There but for the grace of God go I," we may catch ourselves
thinking as we pass someone grotesquely oversize.

In both cases, we seldom think that God may literally figure
into the equation. It's just a figure of speech, we tell ourselves—
but is it? We may have faith in God, but we seldom have faith that
God can and will help us with our overeating. Instead of believing in the power of grace, we believe instead in that dubious
something: our willpower. When willpower fails us, we seldom
think of turning to God for spiritual help.

"I haven't got a prayer of losing weight," Gillian used to say. For
five years she was stubbornly overweight despite trying every diet
that she came across. To see Gillian now, it is difficult to believe
she was ever overweight. She is slim, willowy, and serene. She has
lost weight and found a higher power.

"I lost ten pounds the very first month that I began to include

God in my weight-loss schemes," says Gillian. "I had tried so many other things. It never occurred to me to 'try God'—not until I was genuinely desperate. A friend of mine had gotten sober in Alcoholics Anonymous. I knew that was a spiritually based program. She suggested I try a spiritual solution and I found myself thinking, 'Well, why not?' "

Why not, indeed? I suggested to Gillian that she make her Morning Pages a time when she formally reached out to God for help with the day she had at hand. "Try turning your day over," I suggested. "Try to let go and let God."

Gillian was open-minded enough to try a spiritual solution. She used her Morning Pages to pray, asking for help with the day that lay ahead of her. "Help me to eat clean today," she prayed. "Help me to use food as it is intended to be used. Please give me emotional sobriety. Help me not to act out."

Using her journal, Gillian prayed on the page throughout her day. When a Snack Attack struck, she asked for the grace to weather the cravings. As she prayed, she began to feel new power flowing into her. She had hit upon an unsuspected inner resource that she gradually came to call God.

"I found I wanted to know like-minded others," says Gillian. "A friend—the same one who had gotten sober—suggested that I try Overeaters Anonymous. I found two meetings a week that I liked very much. We had a common problem and we shared a common solution."

Adrienne, an overweight friend of Gillian's, found herself balking at the idea of a spiritual solution. "I couldn't believe God wanted to be bothered with me," she confesses. "I thought God had bigger fish to fry than whether I ever again made it into a size twelve."

I urged Adrienne to experiment a little with the God idea. If God's eye was on the sparrow, might it not also be on her dress size?

"Oh, all right!" fumed Adrienne, and took herself to the page and "turned herself in" to God every morning. "Something's working," she announced two weeks into her new regimen. She was no longer overeating.

I thought the "something working" was God. Adrienne chose to remain an agnostic, but every morning she prayed "just in case." The days of her Clean Eating built up, and her weight slipped down. First she was a size sixteen. Then a fourteen. Then, against her own disbelief, she was once again a twelve. "Maybe God is on my side," she began to joke.

To the members of Overeaters Anonymous, God is no laughing matter. They have tried the spiritual solution, and they know that for them it works. It works for many people without a formal program affiliation, too, although there is a tremendous bond to be found, as Gillian discovered, in sharing with like-minded others.

TASK

Try the Spiritual Solution

Take pen in hand. Setting aside skepticism, write God a letter asking for help with your weight problem. Be detailed and specific about how bad your overeating makes you feel. Ask for guidance and grace. Ask for strength and courage. Ask for good humor as well.

Affirmations

An affirmation is a strong positive statement that something is already so," states spiritual teacher Shakti Gawain. To the un-tutored ear, an affirmation is a positive statement of belief that may sound a little too positive to our skeptical selves.

It is astonishingly difficult to think and speak affirmatively about our weight. The moment we try an affirmative statement, no matter how innocent, we are met with a roar of disbelief from our own subconscious. These objections are what I call blurts. They are very poisonous and must be consciously dismantled. Let us try a simple affirmation: "My body is slender, fit, and beauti-ful." What objections do you hear? You might have heard "My body is fat, flabby, and ugly." Typically the objections we uncover are highly negative and self-hating. Now try it again.

"My body is slender, fit, and beautiful." Now what do you hear? It might be a sarcastic rejoinder like "Oh, yeah? Not lately." Typically our blurts have a sarcastic tone. It helps to remember that sarcasm, from the Greek, means "to cut or tear flesh." In working with affirmations, we are working with the power of our subconscious minds. We are seeking an agreement between our conscious and subconscious selves. We strive to be positive, and when the negatives emerge, we must uproot them like weeds in our garden.

It takes a certain amount of daring to try working with affirmations. We must be willing to stand firm in the face of our subconscious's bluster and bile.

"I thought affirmations were airy-fairy nonsense," says Veronica. "At best, they were simply wishful thinking. At worst, they were delusionary. Then I tried them for thirty days. I was astonished at the difference they made." Working in her journal, Veronica wrote, "My body is slender, fit, and beautiful." She wrote it although she was four dress sizes overweight. She wrote it although her body was untoned. She wrote it although she did not like the image she saw in the mirror. Writing her affirmation daily, Veronica soon sensed its power. She began to eat more lightly. She began to exercise more. Even her posture, a longstanding problem, improved.

The ideal time to work with affirmations is in the morning, just after Morning Pages. Pen in hand, we put our dream on the page: "My body is slender, fit, and beautiful." We listen to our ugly objections as they roar to the surface of our mind. Ignoring their vicious content, we again insist on the positive. "My body is slender, fit, and beautiful." Most of us find there is a particular affirmation that signifies our dreams come true. Affirmations can reflect our highly individual aspirations.

"I have a tiny waist and an hourglass figure."

"I am lean, toned, and vigorous."

"I wear a size eight easily."

"My clothes fit me comfortably and look well."

"My body is trim and muscular."

"My abs are clearly defined."

Affirmations work like an ejector razor blade. We insert the positive as we eject the negative. As we write our affirmations, our blurts lose the power to tyrannize our thinking and our behavior.

"My body is slender, fit, and beautiful" may at first provoke sheer outrage from our subconscious. "What, are you kidding? Have you looked in the mirror lately?" Used repeatedly, this same affirmation works to tame our subconscious. We might hear "Well, at least you're on the path." We might hear "Better than it used to be." We might hear "Keep up your regimen, and these words will be true."

Affirmations declaw the Monster in the Mirror.

"I felt like such a phony, using affirmations," says Judith. "What was I doing, claiming to be thin and beautiful? That's when I realized that affirmations use spiritual law—ask, believe, receive. With my affirmations I was actually asking for healing, and believing in the power of God to make that healing possible. I came to see that it was only a matter of time before I received my answered prayer."

Many of us feel deep-seated resistance as we strive to work with affirmations. We are suddenly too tired to write them. They are too hard, or mere busy work. It sometimes helps to put our resistance on the page in black and white: "My resistance to doing affirmations is . . ." Fill in the blank.

Here are some of the things we heard:

"They'll never work for me."

"I don't have enough faith."

"I'm too distracted."

In using this tool, it is smart to enlist the help of your Body Buddy as a listening ear. Make a phone call to vent your doubts and angers. Then redouble your efforts. Affirmations do work. They are a powerful antidote for our own, often subconscious, negativity.

TASK

Affirm the Affirmative

Take pen in hand. Select an affirmation that reflects your personal fitness ideal. Write your affirmation five times, listening to hear any blurts that may surface. Write down the blurts, and convert any negatives to positives. For example:

"My body is slender, fit, and beautiful."

"Not for long, since you're probably going to miss your workout again."

"I work out regularly. My fitness routine is solid and consistent. My weight goes down as my level of strength goes up. I trust myself and my body."

*My body
is slender
fit + beautiful
My clothes fit me comfortably
and look well — stylish!*

Live and Let Live

Many of us are waiting to live "until." Until we are thinner, until we are fitter, until our clothes fit us better, until we feel better. Our weight has boiled down to "wait." We postpone the adventure of living, and then wonder at our misery, our depression, and our despair. We need to stop waiting.

"I barely left my apartment anymore," recalls Kathleen. "I was embarrassed by what I looked like, and my embarrassment made me self-centered. I imagined being stared at out on the street. I was afraid to venture out."

Kathleen's is not an isolated case. Many of us spend too much time alone and indoors. We told ourselves we will get out "in the spring," "next month," or even "next year."

"I was a prisoner of my own habits," says Jill. "I had a very unfriendly mirror stationed right by my front door. I cannot tell you the number of times I looked in that mirror and decided just to stay home."

"I had to get out to the office," remembers Ralph, "but I was

like a hamster on a wheel. I went from home straight to the office and straight back again. All around me, the city was teeming
with life and adventures, but I was afraid to participate. I was too
fat, I told myself, for other people to accept me. In truth, I was the
one who could not accept me."

For many of us, our first Culinary Artist Date is a radical step.
We are breaking free from our rigid routine and giving our spirit
a taste of adventure. We soon discover that we love these dates and
look forward to them. We are finally beginning to live.

"I live right in Manhattan," says Joan. "Surely it's the adventure
capital of America. My Culinary Artist Dates got me out and
about in the city. At first I was uneasy, but gradually a sense of daring replaced my apprehension. I ventured into ethnic neighborhoods and sampled many foreign cuisines." Joan was interested in
architecture, so she hit on the idea of combining her love of architecture with her walks. An adult education center near her
home offered architectural walks to many parts of the city. Joan
signed up for a series of six walks. "I hope I'll be able to keep up
with everyone," she thought.

Joan did keep up with everyone—in fact, she found her fellow
walkers to be a lively and interesting crew. She began walking
with a man named George, who asked her if she'd like to take in
a movie later in the week. She said she would.

"I had told myself I was too heavy for anyone to be interested
in me, but George seemed to find me interesting despite my reser-
vations. I accepted a movie date, and then a date to hear some live
music. Before I knew it, I had a boyfriend on my hands."

I cannot promise you that if you get out of the house on an

adventure you will wind up with a boyfriend. I can promise you that you will wind up falling in love—with yourself. There is nothing like an adventure to raise your sense of self-worth.

"I was living my life through others," recalls Carolina. "Sidelined myself, I fell into a habit of critiquing those around me. No one could do anything right. I found fault with everything and everybody. 'Mom, you're so negative,' my teenage daughter complained, and she was right."

"The slogan is 'Live and let live,' " I explained to Carolina. "If you are not living enough, it's all too easy not to let live as well." In 12-step terms, we must learn to "put the focus on ourselves." Rather than criticizing the lives of others, we must turn our attention to our own lives, and if those lives feel empty, we must gently fill them with adventures.

"I went to the fabric district," exults Isadora. "I was tired of feeling fat and housebound. I was tired of having no clothes that fit. I'm a good seamstress, and all I needed was to get out my sewing machine and get out of the house. A good fabric store is like a fairyland for me. It is a whole world of possibilities. Even if I buy a plain blue gabardine, I've stopped to stroke aubergine taffeta. I've dreamed a little."

Positive dreams are a knack that many of us lack. Overweight, we find ourselves weighted down by envy of those who are thinner, fitter, and lead more interesting lives. Much to our dismay, we find ourselves focused on others—the fun they are having, the intimacy they seem to be enjoying. We want to live and let live, but we don't know how.

Living begins a day at a time. Each day is a blank canvas. Each day in our Morning Pages we can sketch in some small, even tiny adventure. Adventures build upon adventures. Helen, who was nearly housebound, began by taking herself to the corner Korean greengrocer for fresh flowers. Next she took herself on a crack-of-dawn adventure to her city's flower market. There she bought armloads of flowers at wholesale prices.

"I felt so in the know," she laughs. "Not to mention how lovely my apartment felt filled with flowers and lit by candlelight." If Helen's apartment sounds like the setting for a romantic date, that is an accurate way to describe the process of live and let live. We are learning to woo ourselves, to romance our creative spirits. When we take even the smallest adventure into self-love, further love follows.

TASK

Live and Let Live

Take pen in hand. Number from one to five. List five small adventures you could take. Select the one that sounds most enticing to you. Execute it.

Clean Eating Equals
Clean Living

The problem most overeaters face is that we eat when we're not hungry. We eat when we don't need to eat. We eat because we like eating, but then we hate ourselves because we overate. This brings us to a central question: What can I do instead of eating?

"I was what you might call a grazer," says Mary Lou. "From the time I woke up in the morning until the time I went to bed at night, I ate more or less constantly. Meals blended into snacks, which blended into meals, which blended into snacks again. When I tried Clean Eating, it was a shock to my system. Three meals a day plus two snacks was a lot less than I was accustomed to consuming. Suddenly I had food on my mind and time on my hands. I needed to do something besides eat. The something I chose? Decluttering."

Many of us find that when clarity comes to our food, clarity comes to our mind as well. We experience a sudden craving to put things in order. "I don't need that," we catch ourselves thinking, looking around our bedroom. "And I don't need that, or that, or that."

"I started in my bedroom," says Mary Lou. "I filled a plastic garbage bag with all that I discarded. It was astounding how much sheer volume I could be rid of. There were magazines I had read and magazines I would never read. There were letters I planned to answer and letters I would never answer. My whole room was like a giant bird's nest filled with papers and odds and ends. It was a shock to see the room clean. It had probably been years since I'd seen the top of my desk."

Many of us followed Mary Lou's example, turning to cleaning instead of to food. Starting in the bedroom, we progressed to the public rooms. We often discovered a layer of lived-in rubble.

"My little dog, Charlotte, had more than one hundred toys," confesses Emma. "Many of those toys were chewed beyond repair. I filled an entire garbage bag, and Charlotte still had a plentiful selection remaining."

For many of us, the impulse to toss and discard extends to our closets. There are clothes we do not wear and will never wear again. Some of them are dated, some of them are simply wrong for us. There are, too, clothes that are too small, but if they are otherwise suitable we hold on to them. Shoes are another arena where many of us find we have many surplus pairs that are out of style but still taking up closet space. We bag our excess shoes and are often astonished by their bulk. Suddenly our closets look clean and lean. Our clothes are no longer shoved together. There is room for the new.

"Once I decluttered, I saw all the scuffs and scrapes on my

apartment walls," says Jennifer. "Just how long had I lived in dingy rental white? I wanted some color. In fact, I wanted lots of color. 'What's gotten into you?' my husband asked," Jennifer laughs. "It was really a case of what's not gotten into me. When I stopped overeating, I became conscious of my environment."

Some of us declutter, some of us paint, some of us move our furniture. All of us experience the phenomenon that Clean Eating leads to cleaner living.

"My sofa used to sit like an elephant in the middle of my living room," says Janet. "Three weeks into Morning Pages I moved my sofa along one wall. A week later I added a new rug. A week after that I began a regimen of exercise, using my newly liberated space as a home gym."

You may discover you have an urge to exercise. As you cut back from your overeating to a Clean Eating regimen, you will find your body burning fuel more efficiently. You are no longer sluggish and hungover in the mornings. Midafternoon finds you filled with energy instead of needing a nap. As you move room to room through your house, your new energies find focus after focus. You take time to mend the torn throw pillow. You take time to scrub the scuffed doorjambs. You even take time to sort and organize your bookcases. Once again you are astonished by the sheer amount you can discard.

"I had a very successful garage sale," brags Erin. "I earned back dollars for what I discarded. My goal was to earn enough for a new living room rug. I wanted to do yoga."

Erin got her new rug, and she got addicted—happily—to a series of yoga tapes. Eating clean and exercising daily, she lost twenty pounds, but more important, lost inches.

"Nothing fit me anymore," Erin laughs. "Or, to put it differently, everything fit me. I looked good in styles I never dreamed I could carry off."

Clean Eating can lead to a transformation, first of your living space, and then of your life.

TASK

Clean Something

Take pen in hand. Number from one to five. List five areas of your household that could benefit from your focused attention. Cleanliness is next to godliness. Clean something.

Do Something Else

Although we seldom look at it squarely, food is, for many of us, the great obsession. We are always eating, or about to eat, or recovering from eating. Food is our food for thought. We plan special treats for ourselves, even though those treats are treating ourselves badly. One way or another, food is always on our mind. Perhaps we count points in Weight Watchers. Perhaps we count calories. What we can count on, regardless, is that we will overeat.

"Clean Eating is addictive, thank God," says Jaime. "It took me about a week to get hooked, but once I did, I never wanted to look back."

Clean Eating is structured eating. One of the first results of Clean Eating is time. We no longer spend our time on food. We know what we're going to eat and when we're going to eat. Our mind is freed to think of other things. So we need to know what to do with our time.

"I finally began my novel," says Rosemary, who had dreamed for years of writing. "Suddenly I had time. When I wasn't thinking about food, I began thinking about other things—and other characters besides myself."

Lizzie, a visual artist, turned to sculpture to celebrate. "It was Christmas, and instead of baking Christmas cookies I made a fifteen-foot-tall reindeer. A friend of mine told the president of our bank, who came to look at it and bought it outright for his lobby. Now I'm working on Valentine's Day. . . ."

Our newly liberated creativity can lead us into exciting adventures. Some of us turn to fine arts, some of us turn to crafts. Some of us turn to new adventures in the kitchen. No longer addicted to comfort foods, we begin to create meals that are both legal and satisfying. Bookstores are filled with low-cal cookbooks containing low-calorie recipes and most of them are delicious. We stir up a pot of ratatouille. We stir things up generally.

At about the three-week mark, after cleaning her house like a whirling dervish, my friend Alice began writing a children's book. Not about to be outdone, I cleaned my house too. Then I found myself in my kitchen, chopping vegetables. My new obsession became the perfect vegetable soup.

Immersed in our new creative projects, who wants to overeat and spoil it all? Robert, once pudgy but now filled with energy, auditioned for a new musical—and got the part. During rehearsals he lost an additional eight pounds.

Whether we are cooking up pots of soup or the plots for our novels, many of us discover our creativity bubbling over. Suddenly we have the time and impulse for all sorts of projects. We design our own Christmas cards. We make homemade valentines. Our children discover in us willing co-conspirators for their special homework assignments. Suddenly we have time for the papier-mâché monster, the bas-relief map of our home state. Costumes for Halloween? No problem.

Freed from our compulsive eating, the world around us becomes a new and more vivid place. Was it always so beautiful? we wonder. We begin to sketch, paint, and photograph with a vengeance. The world is a thing of beauty, and we are citizens of the world. When we are no longer narrowly focused on our eating, our interests broaden. We subscribe to new magazines and join museums. We get out to galleries and go on garden tours. There are so many things to do other than eat.

"I not only gained a new body, I gained a new life," says Claire.

Many of us feel we have gained new lives. We even feel we have gained new personalities.

"I am the woman I always wanted to be," says Allison. "I'm healthy, fit, trim, and adventurous. I tried the tools with skepticism, but now I've written myself a happy ending."

TASK

Write Yourself a Happy Ending

Take pen in hand. Make a written inventory of yourself—the ways that you have changed and the ways you hope to continue to change.

One of the first results of successful Clean Eating is a

shift in clarity. When we overeat, we blunt our perceptions. When we eat clean, we sharpen them. Take pen in hand again. Ask yourself these three questions:

1. What do I need to know?
2. What do I need to accept?
3. What do I need to change?

Pose each question, and listen to the answer that bubbles up from within you. These questions constitute a spot-check inventory. Use them at regular intervals.

Epilogue:
Staying the Distance

*S*ome people plunge into the Writing Diet wholeheartedly, find it comfortable, and stick to it with relative ease. Others, myself included here, start the diet, do well, then stray a bit and have to start over. It is my experience that starting over is the trick to success.

"It's progress that counts," says Marilyn, who has started over several times. "I used to get so discouraged that I would figure, 'What's the use?' and keep right on eating. I told myself things like 'A binge has to run its course.' Working with the tools, especially journaling, I have learned I can interrupt a binge and start over anytime."

Perseverance is what pays off in the long run. While we may still crave sudden and dramatic weight loss, the kind you read about in the tabloids, we have to learn to content ourselves with gradual and healthy weight loss, the kind you do not often read about. I am down about fifteen pounds, aiming at twenty, and an ounce at a time I believe I will get there. My looser clothes tell me that I will.

Annette, a Weight Watchers leader, puts her experience this

way: "I like to see people lose a pound—even half a pound—a week. That seems slow, but it adds up quickly. When people lose weight more rapidly, they often binge and pile it right back on. No, I have to say 'Easy does it' is what works."

While "Easy does it" is what works, sometimes we stop working it. It's the holiday season and we just can't resist a handful of cookies and a slab of peppermint bark. What to do, now that we've "done it"?

"Drink water," says Annette.

"Drink water," echoes Sara Ryba.

Poisoned by a binge, we can turn to water, and we can pick up our tool kit to start again. We might use journaling, keeping a meticulous food log. We might use the four questions. Pen in hand, it is difficult to keep acting out.

Bottom line, starting over is the key to eventual success. "I needed to learn to say 'oops!'" says Patricia, "and get right back on the horse. I needed to tell myself that a slip was just a slip and not a catastrophic fall. In short, I needed to learn to be more self-loving, and to gently put myself back on track as soon as possible."

Our goal is to establish new eating habits, and new eating habits take time to root. Little by little, one day at a time, we improve. We use our four questions and gradually they become an ingrained part of our consciousness. "Am I really hungry?" we learn to ask, and when the answer is no, but we still feel a Snack Attack, we learn to dig deeper, asking ourselves not only "What do I want to eat?" but also "What's eating me?" The habit of healthy introspection that we establish through the use of our journal often creates a ripple effect in our life as a whole.

"'You're so much more calm,' people tell me," says Paula. And she is more calm. Writing has become a way of life for her. When she slips up, she simply starts over. She has lost twenty pounds and is confident she will lose the final ten to reach her goal weight. "I needed to learn to get back on the bicycle. I was so dramatic that every time I relapsed, I went into an emotional spiral. I made life miserable for my husband and my family."

Making a drama out of a relapse sets you up to relapse further still. A small slip on a chocolate chip cookie becomes the large slip on a generous slice of chocolate mousse cake. By learning to say "oops" instead of "what a catastrophe!" you train yourself to start over again immediately rather than finish your bender.

Once I learned to start over, I became connected to the solution rather than to the problem. The solution always says, "Start now." The problem always says, "Not just yet." My Morning Pages and my journal always told me that the time to start was right now. No more procrastinating. No more telling myself "someday."

This book has been a year in the writing. That's four twelve-week creativity cycles. During that time I've found myself, like my students, slowly and gradually slimming down. At first it was very difficult. I felt that my medication was slowing my metabolism to a near standstill. I believed that no matter what I ate, or didn't eat, I packed on pounds. But at the suggestion of my Morning Pages, I stayed consistent on my food plan, I recommitted to my exercise regimen, and the Writing Diet really began to work for me. Ounces gave way to pounds. Sizes slipped away. I started at a size sixteen and am now a ten.

At this writing I am still pudgier than I would like to be, but I am far slimmer than I was. My consciousness around food has shifted. My refrigerator is now stocked with tasty and healthful foods. Best of all, my own attitudes have undergone a sea change. I start each day determined to do well, and if I slip, I start over. I have the support of my tools and my Body Buddy to keep me on track. Furthermore, I have a heightened sense of conscious contact with my Higher Power. My intuition has deepened, and my spiritual life and creative life are more satisfying. It is my hope that the same gentle revolution will happen for you.

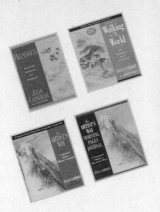
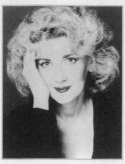
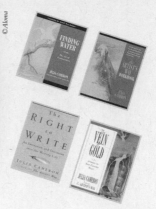

To order call 1-800-788-6262 or visit our website at www.penguin.com

The Artist's Way
ISBN 978-1-58542-147-3 (tenth anniversary hardcover edition)
ISBN 978-1-58542-146-6 (tenth anniversary trade paper edition)
ISBN 978-0-87477-852-6 (audio, cassettes)
ISBN 978-0-14-305825-0 (audio, CDs)

The Complete Artist's Way
ISBN 978-1-58542-630-0 (hardcover)

The Writing Diet
ISBN 978-1-58542-571-6 (hardcover)
ISBN 978-1-58542-698-0 (trade paper)

Prayers to the Great Creator
ISBN 978-1-58542-682-9 (hardcover)

Walking in This World
ISBN 978-1-58542-261-6 (trade paper)

Finding Water
ISBN 978-1-58542-463-4 (hardcover)

The Vein of Gold
ISBN 978-0-87477-879-3 (trade paper)

The Right to Write
ISBN 978-1-58542-009-4 (trade paper)

The Sound of Paper
ISBN 978-1-58542-354-5 (trade paper)

Floor Sample: A Creative Memoir
ISBN 978-1-58542-494-8 (hardcover)

Answered Prayers
ISBN 978-1-58542-351-4 (trade paper)

Heart Steps
ISBN 978-0-87477-899-1 (hardcover)

Blessings
ISBN 978-0-87477-906-6 (trade paper)

Transitions
ISBN 978-0-87477-995-0 (trade paper)

Prayers from a Nonbeliever
ISBN 978-1-58542-213-5 (hardcover)

Letters to a Young Artist
ISBN 978-1-58542-409-2 (hardcover)

How to Avoid Making Art (or Anything Else You Enjoy)
Illustrated by Elizabeth Cameron
ISBN 978-1-58542-438-2 (trade paper)

The Artist's Way Workbook
ISBN 978-1-58542-533-4 (trade paper)

The Artist's Way Morning Pages Journal
ISBN 978-0-87477-886-1 (trade paper)

The Artist's Date Book
Illustrated by Elizabeth Cameron
ISBN 978-0-87477-653-9 (trade paper)

God Is No Laughing Matter
ISBN 978-1-58542-128-2 (trade paper)

Inspirations: Meditations from The Artist's Way
ISBN 978-1-58542-102-2 (trade paper)

The Writer's Life: Insights from The Right to Write
ISBN 978-1-58542-103-9 (trade paper)